T0156609

Prevent, Detect and Reverse Heart Disease

MOHAMED SHALABY, M.D.

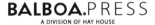
BALBOA.PRESS
A DIVISION OF HAY HOUSE

Balboa Press books may be ordered through booksellers or by contacting:

Balboa Press
A Division of Hay House
1663 Liberty Drive
Bloomington, IN 47403
www.balboapress.com
844-682-1282

Print information available on the last page.

ISBN: 978-1-9822-5908-2 (sc)
ISBN: 978-1-9822-5909-9 (e)

Balboa Press rev. date: 11/28/2020

CONTENTS

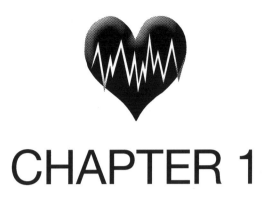

CHAPTER 1

Introduction

HEART DISEASE IS THE NUMBER-ONE cause of death around the world and in the United States. It accounts for almost 380,000 American deaths a year—that's about one in six—according to the American Heart Association's *Heart Disease and Stroke Statistical Update 2014*. Indeed, about 2,150 Americans die every day from some form of heart disease, one every forty seconds. The American Heart Association estimates that the disease costs Americans $315.4 billion a year, including health expenses and lost productivity.

When you add in heart disease, stroke, and other cardiovascular diseases, that figure more than doubles. In 2010, for instance, the American Heart Association reported that 787,000 Americans died of heart disease; that's one in three deaths—nearly one death every minute and a half, just in the United States.

These statistics make heart disease sound inevitable, like tax increases and winter snowstorms. And, in fact, there are some risk factors that you can't control: age, gender, race, and family history.

The good news is that over the past ten years, when the statistics have been available, the death rate from heart disease has fallen about 39 percent and the number of stroke-related deaths has decreased by roughly 23 percent, according to the American Heart Association. Of course, there's still plenty of room for improvement.

Lifestyle changes go a long way to staving off heart disease and repairing some or much of the damage after it has occurred. Probably the biggest items on the list are not smoking, keeping active, eating healthy, maintaining a suitable body weight, and controlling your blood-pressure and blood-sugar levels.

The Most Common Types of Heart Disease

The heart is a complex and delicate mechanism, so it's no wonder things can go wrong with it. There are many different kinds of heart disease. Here is a brief list of the most common types:

Atherosclerosis. Also known as hardening of the arteries, atherosclerosis happens when plaque builds up in the walls of the arteries and makes it hard for the blood to flow properly.

Coronary Artery Disease (CAD). CAD happens when atherosclerosis hits a coronary artery and can lead to coronary heart disease, which can lead to angina (chest pain or discomfort) or a heart attack. CAD is the most common type of heart disease and the number-one cause of death in the United States.

Heart Attack. Heart attacks, also known as myocardial infarctions (MIs), affect more than a million Americans every year. They occur when the heart isn't getting enough oxygen-rich blood to function.

Heart Failure. When you hear "heart failure," you think it means that the heart has stopped working altogether. But it really means that the heart isn't working as well as it should

Arrhythmia. Arrhythmia means that your heart doesn't beat regularly. Sometimes, this lack of rhythm is as innocuous as the guy who just can't tap his foot in time to the music, but other times it can mean that the lungs, brain, and other body organs aren't getting as much blood as they should.

Warning Signs

Heart disease, as with any other illness, is easiest to treat if caught early. But early heart disease often doesn't have symptoms, or it has symptoms that are barely noticeable—especially in older adults, who may have a lot going on with their bodies. That's why regular doctor checkups are key. Your doctor may send you to a cardiologist, who specializes in heart issues.

One of the reasons heart disease is so deadly is that people don't seek help when they have symptoms. Sure, if someone grabs his or her chest and falls over, people rush to help. If someone stops breathing, people whip out their phones and dial 911. But many of the symptoms of heart disease are a little more subtle than that.

The National Institutes of Health's Institute on Aging recommends talking to your doctor about any of these symptoms, which could indicate heart problems:

- Pain in the shoulders, arms, neck, jaw, or back
- Shortness of breath when active or at rest
- Chest pain during physical activity that gets better when you rest
- Lightheadedness
- Dizziness
- Confusion
- Headaches
- Cold sweats
- Nausea or vomiting
- Getting easily tired or fatigued
- Swelling in the ankles, feet, legs, stomach, or neck
- Difficulty exercising or being physically active
- Experiencing problems doing your normal activities

The American Heart Association lists warning signs of specific heart conditions:

Heart Attack

- Chest discomfort
- Discomfort in other parts of the upper body
- Shortness of breath

Stroke

- Face drooping
- Arm weakness
- Difficulty with speech

Cardiac Arrest

- Sudden loss of responsiveness
- Abnormal breathing

If you experience any of these signs—or if anyone around you does—call your doctor or dial 911.

Important Points

- Heart disease is the number-one killer in the United States. It accounts for one out of every six deaths in this country.
- The most common types are atherosclerosis, CAD, heart attack, heart failure, and arrhythmia.
- There are a range of symptoms and warning signs. Women especially are less likely to experience the characteristic pain—like an elephant sitting on your chest—and more likely to have chest pain that isn't quite so extreme, but should still be checked out.
- If you feel like you're having a heart attack or think a friend or family member is having one, call 911.

CHAPTER 2

Risk Factors

PREDICTING HEART DISEASE ISN'T AS simple as we all wish it was. There are a variety of major contributors to the risk of heart disease, as well as a host of minor ones. And, unfortunately, some of the risk factors for heart disease are completely out of your control. The good news, though, is that there are a number of factors you can control, and making certain lifestyle choices can cut your risk of heart disease by as much as 82 percent, according to a Harvard University study.

Let's take a look at some of the factors.

Factors That Are Out of Your Control

There's nothing you can do about certain issues. Unless you've figured out how to change your age, gender, race, or family history, there's not much you can do to counteract the effects of these issues on your heart health.

But if you know you're at increased risk for heart disease, you *can* keep an eye out for the symptoms and make lifestyle changes to decrease your risk. You can also make sure your doctor monitors your health regularly—typically once a year—to catch any potential problems as early as possible.

Here are the immutable risk factors:

Age. They say you're only as old as you feel; part of how you feel, though, has to do with how your heart is doing. Risk factors that lead to heart disease develop slowly over time, according to the American College of Cardiology. They can take years and even decades to develop. According to the American Heart Association, about 82 percent of people who die of coronary heart disease are at least sixty-five years of age.

The risk of atrial fibrillation (AFib) increases with age too; AFib is a type of arrhythmia that increases the risk of stroke or heart failure. We don't want to suggest that you avoid getting older, only that you realize your risk increases and lifestyle changes become increasingly important as you age.

Gender. Men are more likely to have heart attacks than women, and they have them at younger ages, according to the American Heart Association. Women's risk of heart disease rises after menopause, but it still doesn't catch up with men's risk. The risk of atrial fibrillation increases with age, but men tend to develop AFib at age sixty-seven, whereas women are more likely to run into trouble at age seventy-five. Older women who have heart attacks are more likely to die within a few weeks than are older men.

However, since 1984, more females than males have died of cardiovascular disease. Although the particulars may vary between men and women, heart health is essential for everyone.

Race. African Americans, Mexican Americans, Native Americans, Native Hawaiians, and some Asian Americans have higher rates of heart disease than white Americans, according to the American Heart Association. African Americans have more severe blood pressure; in fact, nearly half of all African Americans have some sort of heart disease (49 percent of women and 44 percent of men), whereas the other racial minority groups have higher rates of obesity and diabetes than do white Americans.

African Americans: In 2010, heart disease caused the deaths of 46,266 African American males and 49,977 African American females. Between the 1990s and 2005, fewer whites had strokes, but there was no change among blacks. African American children are more likely to be obese than the general population; according to the American Heart Association, about 31.8 percent of all children ages two to nineteen are overweight or obese, but the rates among non-Hispanic black children are 36.9 percent for boys and 41.3 percent for girls. And 44 percent of African Americans have high blood pressure, which is one of the highest rates of any population in the world.

Hispanic Americans: More than a third of Mexican American men (33.4 percent) have had cardiovascular disease; the rate among Mexican American women is slightly lower: 30.7 percent. Mexican Americans are more likely to have intracerebral hemorrhage and subarachnoid hemorrhage than are non-Hispanic whites. Puerto Rican Americans had the highest hypertension-related death rate among all Hispanic groups, whereas Cuban Americans had the lowest.

Native Americans: Obesity is a big issue here; nationally, about 20 percent of all children are obese, but the figure is 31 percent for Native American children. However, diabetes isn't as much of a concern among kids ages ten to nineteen, comparatively speaking; both Native Americans and Asian/Pacific Islanders have lower rates of diabetes than do white youth.

Asian Americans: Asian and Pacific Islander adults are less likely to have cardiovascular disease than the US population as a whole. They are also much less likely to be obese than the rest of the population. Korean Americans are two to three times as likely to smoke as Japanese Americans, Asian Indians, or Chinese Americans. Asian Indians are more than twice as likely to have diabetes as are Japanese Americans or Chinese Americans.

Family History. Heart disease: it's all in the family. If either of your parents had heart disease, you have a greater chance of getting it as well. In fact, the American Heart Association notes that people with a strong family history of heart disease also have one or more other risk factors. But, again, this does not mean that you will definitely get heart disease—only that you have to be more careful than people without this risk factor.

Other Standard Factors

Fortunately, there are some heart-disease risk factors that you can do something about. Lifestyle changes can do a lot to reduce your risk and even repair some or most of the damage of heart disease. Here are the major factors:

High Blood Pressure or Hypertension. High blood pressure happens when the force of blood against the artery walls is too high. This pressure causes the heart muscle to thicken and become stiffer, which, in turn, forces the heart to work harder to achieve the same results. Usually, high blood pressure causes no symptoms that you can detect—doctors call it the "silent killer" for this very reason; you don't know it's lurking, but if left uncontrolled, high blood pressure increases the risk for heart attack and stroke.

Cholesterol. Cholesterol is a waxy, fatlike substance that's found in all body cells. It's not inherently bad; our body needs some cholesterol to make hormones, vitamin D, and various substances to help digest food. But it's possible too much of a good thing. If you have too much cholesterol in your blood, plaque builds up on your artery walls. As your cholesterol level rises, so does the risk of heart disease. Basically, you want your total cholesterol to be less than 180 mg/dl, including both high-density lipoprotein (HDL, often called "good" cholesterol) and low-density lipoprotein (LDL, or "bad" cholesterol).

Obesity. People with excess body weight, especially around the waist, are more likely to develop heart disease even if they have no other risk factors. That's because obesity tends to raise the blood pressure, cholesterol level, triglycerides level, and chances of diabetes, all of which then force the heart to work harder to keep the body going. According to the American College of Cardiology, abdominal obesity means having a waist circumference greater than forty inches for a man or thirty-five inches for a woman.

Diabetes. Diabetes is a disease where your blood-sugar level (glucose) is too high. In fact, people who have type 2 diabetes, where the body's cells don't use insulin properly, have the same risk of heart attack and dying from heart disease as people who've already had heart attacks. Even when your glucose levels are under control, there is still an increased chance of heart disease. According to the American Heart Association, more than half (65 percent or more) of people with diabetes die of some form of heart or blood vessel disease.

Smoking. These days, most people know that smoking isn't exactly a health-conscious activity. Smoking harms just about every part of the body, including the heart and blood vessels. It causes about one in five deaths every year in the United States. A smoker has between two and four times as great a chance of developing heart disease as a nonsmoker. The good news is that quitting smoking can help decrease the risk surprisingly quickly.

Other Potential Risk Factors

We're getting better and better at predicting risk for heart disease, with researchers finding new and exciting indicators. The more you know—and the sooner you know it—the better your chances are of fixing the situation and avoiding heart disease. Here are some of the state-of-the-art detectors of risk factors.

C-reactive Protein (CRP). While we know that high cholesterol causes heart disease, only about half the people who have heart attacks have high cholesterol, according to Harvard Medical School, which makes it harder to predict a person's risk. Healthy people have only very small amounts of CRP in their bloodstream; once there's an injury of some sort, such as heart disease, the liver starts churning out extra CRP to help repair the damage.

Studies have found that as the CRP level rises, so does the risk of having—or dying from—a heart attack, stroke, or other cardiovascular problem. So some physicians have begun looking into checking CRP levels as a way to predict risk for heart disease.

Homocysteine. Homocysteine is an amino acid typically found in blood. Studies have shown that high levels of it can boost the risk of heart disease. This observation is particularly relevant for women, because their homocysteine levels tend to rise after menopause.

According to the American Heart Association, there has been no causal link between homocysteine and heart disease. The National Institutes of Health suggests that it may be possible to lower elevated levels of homocysteine by getting plenty of folic acid and vitamins B_6 and B_{12} in your diet.

Cholesterol Subfractions. According to the Mayo Clinic website, Lp(a) protein, or lipoprotein (a), is a type of LDL ("bad") cholesterol. This lipoprotein may make it easier for blood clots to form, though it is unclear how much risk it adds to the individual. Your Lp(a) level is determined by your genes and generally isn't affected by lifestyle. The National Institutes of Health suggests that niacin, a cholesterol-lowering drug, may lower Lp(a) levels in women.

Coronary Calcium. Calcium can accumulate in arteries, making them stiffer and potentially blocking the supply of blood to the heart. As a result, the heart must work harder, which can lead to high blood pressure, angina (chest pain), and heart failure. Although calcium doesn't actually do any harm to the heart, if someone has high coronary calcium, it can indicate the presence of advanced plaques. According to Harvard Medical School, calcium detection may help in diagnosing atherosclerosis, but heart disease cannot be treated by removing calcium.

Plaque Detection. The presence of atherosclerotic plaque in the thoracic aorta appears to indicate increased risk of heart disease, according to a 1993 article in a National Institutes of Health study, which indicated that the approach "warrants further investigation."

All of this information about heart-disease risk allows us to take stock of our situation and make the appropriate lifestyle changes to decrease our risk. Bear in mind, though, that having even one risk factor for heart disease is concerning. And each additional risk factor increases your chances of developing heart disease; risk factors tend to "gang up" and worsen each other's effects. It's important to take heart-disease risk seriously—and do something about it.

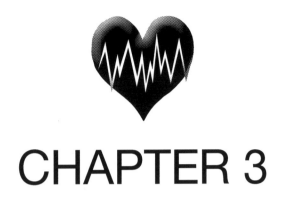

CHAPTER 3

Heart Disease in Special Populations

MOST OF WHAT YOU READ in newspapers and magazines about heart health focuses on older men. But, eart health is an issue for everyone.

Women and young people, especially athletes, are often forgotten or ignored in this discussion, and their symptoms or telltale signs are often dismissed. In addition, sometimes the symptoms women experience are a little different than what we see in men. Unfortunately, while women and young people are sitting around wondering whether to contact a doctor, damage is happening. It is important for everyone to pay attention to heart health. In this chapter, we will take a closer look at these two special populations.

Women's Heart Health

Women are becoming more and more aware of the dangers of heart disease, according to a 2013 American Heart Association study. But even so, younger women and minorities aren't as aware as they ought to be.

Unfortunately, women's risk of heart disease is quite high. According to the National Institutes of Health,

+   one in four women in the United States dies of heart disease, while one in thirty dies of breast cancer;

- almost one in four American women (23 percent) dies within a year after having a heart attack; and

- within six years of having a heart attack, about 46 percent of women in the United States become disabled with heart failure. Two-thirds of women who have a heart attack fail to make a full recovery.

Perhaps most surprisingly, according to the American Heart Association, since 1984, more women than men have died each year from heart disease. Part of the problem may be that women often experience less dramatic symptoms than men: they're more likely to have general fatigue and a flu-like discomfort and no chest pain at all. So they may wait longer than men to seek medical help.

In fact, women tend to wait longer than men before getting help for a possible heart attack. One study found that women wait an average of twenty-two minutes longer than men before they go to the hospital. Some say they don't want to bother anyone, especially in case their symptoms turn out to be a false alarm.

However, autopsy reports show that women who die of heart attacks have completely different experiences than men. Women are much more likely than men to have coronary microvascular disease (MVD), which affects the tiny coronary arteries.

In the 1970s, a large National Institutes of Health research study on the heart was the first to include women. Interestingly, the results were puzzling, and researchers concluded that women had a much lower incidence of heart disease than men. Doctors continued treating women with the same procedures as men; however, women tended to have much worse outcomes. By the year 2000, the rates had increased to the point where 60,000 more women were dying of heart disease than men.

Often, the symptoms signaling a heart attack in women are somewhat different than they are for men. And since the media tends to focus on men's symptoms, many women aren't aware of this. Women should know that they are mostly likely to experience these symptoms:

- Discomfort or pressure in the chest
- Pain in the arms, upper back, neck, jaw, or stomach
- Nausea or vomiting
- Trouble breathing

+ Breaking out in a cold sweat
+ Dizziness or lightheadedness
+ Inability to sleep
+ Unusual fatigue
+ Clammy skin

Some women may not experience all of these symptoms; they may have just a few. When in doubt, though, dial 911.

Conditions That Affect Women More Than Men

Heart disease is, for the most part, an equal-opportunity offender. However, some types of heart disease affect women more than men. That's not to say that men are off the hook—only that women need to be particularly aware of these conditions. These conditions have not been studied as thoroughly as the types of heart disease already discussed.

Coronary Microvascular Disease (MVD): Coronary MVD operates a little differently than coronary artery disease. Rather than affecting the major arteries, coronary MVD works on the walls and inner lining of the body's tiny coronary arteries. This damage leads to spasms in the blood vessels, which blocks blood flow.

Scientists speculate that the drop in hormone levels that women experience after menopause makes them more vulnerable. Tests designed to assess risk of coronary heart disease do not predict coronary MVD because they look for blockages in the large coronary arteries; but coronary MVD affects the smaller ones, so the large ones appear to be perfectly healthy.

The symptoms of coronary MVD are also slightly different than those for coronary artery disease. Women with coronary MVD often have angina (a pain or uncomfortable feeling in the chest) that usually lasts for more than ten minutes—and can last for more than thirty minutes. Other symptoms include the following:

+ Shortness of breath
+ Sleep problems
+ Fatigue
+ Lack of energy

Interestingly, these symptoms usually appear during normal daily activities and at times of mental stress, but they are less apt to show up during physical exertion.

Coronary MVD is also called cardiac syndrome X and nonobstructive coronary heart disease.

Broken Heart Syndrome: If an emotional time leaves you feeling like your heart is breaking, you may be right.

A relatively recently discovered phenomenon, broken heart syndrome, occurs when extreme emotional distress leads to severe, though often short-term, heart-muscle failure. It presents as sudden, intense chest pain and shortness of breath. What's going on is that part of your heart is temporarily enlarging and not pumping properly. This syndrome is often misdiagnosed as a heart attack.

The good news is that women who have experienced it show no sign of blocked arteries and usually have a full and quick recovery, though sometimes it can be fatal. Women who've experienced broken heart syndrome are not at risk for recurrence.

Broken heart syndrome is also called stress-induced cardiomyopathy or takotsubo cardiomyopathy.

Gender Differences in Risk Factors

Men and women share many of the risk factors for heart disease, but there are some differences:

Smoking: While smoking isn't a good idea for anyone, women who smoke increase their risk of heart disease even more than men do. In addition, women who smoke and take birth control pills have an extra added risk for heart disease.

Cholesterol: For men, the danger sign is LDL above 130 mg/dl. For women, the alarm bell goes off when they have levels of HDL that are below 50 mg/dl or triglyceride levels over 150 mg/dl.

Blood Pressure: Up to age forty-five, men are more likely than women to have high blood pressure. In middle age, though, women start catching up. By age seventy, women typically have higher blood pressure than men.

Diabetes: Having diabetes increases the risk of heart disease for both men and women, but the danger is greater for women. Men's risk rises by 60 percent if they have diabetes; women's risk doubles.

Pregnancy: Women have a greater risk of heart disease during pregnancy than otherwise, even among women with no history of heart disease. The risk lasts until about twelve weeks after delivery.

Atrial Fibrillation (. Someone with AFib has an irregular heartbeat. The risk of atrial fibrillation increases with age, but men tend to develop AFib at age sixty-seven, whereas women are more likely to run into trouble at age seventy-five. Older women who have heart attacks are more likely to die within a few weeks than older men.

Also, women experience more AFib symptoms than men: palpitations (40 percent in women, 27 percent in men); dizziness (23 percent in women, 19 percent in men); fatigue (28 percent in women, 25 percent in men); and chest tightness/discomfort (11 percent in women, 8 percent in men). In addition, women with AFib have a higher risk of stroke and a lower quality of life, according to the American College of Cardiology.

Inflammation: Women are more likely than men to suffer from chronic inflammation due to atherosclerotic plaque. This condition makes the artery more likely to rupture, which can cause a heart attack.

Metabolic Syndrome: It's the name for a group of risk factors that raises the risk of heart disease. The risk factors for this syndrome are abdominal obesity, high blood pressure, high triglycerides, low HDL cholesterol, and high blood sugar/insulin resistance. Having any three of these risk factors boosts the risk of heart disease. A large waist circumference–high triglyceride combo is particularly concerning for women.

African American and Mexican American women experiencing metabolic syndrome have a greater chance of heart disease than men of the same racial groups, according to the National Heart, Lung, and Blood Institute. The rates are about the same among white women and men.

Additional Risk Factors for Women

Efforts to regulate or control women's hormones and reproductive capacities can lead to unanticipated problems when it comes to matters of the heart. Specifically, hormone replacement therapy and birth control pills can increase women's risk of heart disease.

Hormone Replacement Therapy (HRT): At one point, we thought that hormone treatment was sort of a magic wand for the ills of menopause: it could ward off heart disease, osteoporosis, and cancer, while improving women's quality of life (such as improving hot flashes). But we've found that hormone treatment can actually increase the chances of heart disease.

But this increased risk varies by age. Studies show that older women—ages sixty to seventy-nine—taking estrogen are not protected against heart disease, but it might be helpful among women ages fifty to fifty-nine. Talk with your doctor, and weigh the risks with the benefits.

Birth Control Pills: Women who use high-dosage birth control pills are more likely to have clots in their blood vessels, which leads to an increased chance of heart attack or stroke. Taking the pill can also worsen the effects of risk factors like smoking, high blood pressure, diabetes, high blood cholesterol, and being overweight.

Researchers have only looked at the effect of high-dosage birth control pills; we don't know what happens if you're taking low-dosage pills. Again, it's important to talk with your doctor and think about benefit versus risk.

For women, it's important to know the risk of heart disease. The more risk factors women have, the greater the chance of developing problems.

The next step is to *use* this knowledge: Even if you have several risk factors, you can adopt a healthier lifestyle and cut your chances of having a heart attack or stroke. It's never too late, or too early, to make important changes.

Young People and Heart Disease

Young people, especially athletes, often think they're invincible, with no chance of having heart disease (as well as other conditions). Although heart disease does, in fact, affect older people more than younger ones—the average age of a person with heart disease is sixty-two—everyone is vulnerable.

As many as 4 percent to 10 percent of all heart attacks occur before age forty-five—mostly striking males. Don't ignore the warning symptoms just because you think you are "too young" to have heart disease.

Some conditions, in fact, tend to target younger people more often. Congenital heart disease, congenital coronary anomalies, mitral valve prolapse, and hypertrophic cardiomyopathy are some of the prime culprits in young heart patients.

Probably the most concerning aspect of heart disease in young people is that because no one expects these individuals to have coronary problems, people usually ignore any warning symptoms or risk factors. So it is particularly important to know about these conditions.

Congenital Heart Disease

This term refers to any abnormalities in the heart that are present at birth. They affect the normal flow of blood through the heart and can include problems with the following:

+ The heart's interior walls
+ Valves inside the heart
+ Arteries and veins that carry blood to the heart or around the body

Some people experience symptoms at birth, others as children, still others as adults, and some lucky people don't experience any symptoms at all. Symptoms typically include shortness of breath and difficulty exercising.

Usually, doctors detect congenital heart disease when they hear an unusual heart sound, called a murmur, as they listen to the heart. They may then order further testing.

Treatment depends on how severe the condition is. Some mild heart defects don't require any treatment, whereas others can be treated with medications or surgery. Most adults with congenital heart disease are monitored by a heart specialist throughout their lives.

Congenital Coronary Anomalies (CCA)

A CCA, which is present at birth, means there is a defect in one or more of the coronary arteries. This defect can reduce the amount of oxygen and nutrients that the heart receives, which impairs its functioning.

Although CCA is very rare it can be dangerous. It is the second-leading cause of death in young athletes; between 15 percent and 34 percent of young people who experience sudden cardiac death are later found to have a CCA.

Most people with CCA have no symptoms. Among those who do experience symptoms, babies and children may have

- breathing problems;
- pale skin;
- poor feeding; and
- sweating.

Teens and adults with CCA may experience

- fainting during strenuous exercise;
- shortness of breath at rest or during exercise;
- fatigue; and
- chest pain at rest or during exercise.

Mitral Valve Prolapse (MVP)

This condition is generally harmless. It happens when the two flaps of the heart's mitral valve do not close smoothly or evenly. Sometimes, the prolapsed valve allows a little blood to leak backward, which could cause a heart murmur.

There usually aren't any symptoms, so doctors typically find it when they listen to the heart. Occasionally, though, people do experience these symptoms:

- Chest pain
- Dizziness
- Fatigue
- Sensation of feeling the heart beat
- Shortness of breath with activity or when lying flat

People with MVP rarely experience problems, but you should let your doctor decide about your particular situation. At one point, people with MVP routinely took antibiotics before dental examinations and procedures, but the American Heart Association no longer recommends this.

MVP, which affects 2 percent to 3 percent of the population, is also known as click-murmur syndrome, Barlow's syndrome, and floppy valve syndrome.

Hypertrophic Cardiomyopathy (HCM)

HCM happens when the heart muscle—most often, only one part of the organ—becomes thick. This thickening makes the heart work harder to pump blood, and it can also make it more difficult for the heart to relax and fill with blood.

HCM is common, affecting about one out of every five hundred people, and hits men and women of all ages. Young people often have a more severe form of the condition, and it is a common cause of sudden cardiac arrest in young people, including young athletes.

Some people have no symptoms, whereas others experience one or more of the following symptoms:

- Chest pain
- Dizziness
- Fainting, especially during exercise
- Fatigue
- Lightheadedness, especially with or after activity or exercise
- Sensation of feeling the heart beat
- Shortness of breath with activity or after lying down (or after being asleep for a while)

HCM is also called asymmetric septal hypertrophy, familial hypertrophic cardiomyopathy, hypertrophic nonobstructive cardiomyopathy, hypertrophic obstructive cardiomyopathy, and idiopathic hypertrophic subaortic stenosis (IHSS).

Atherosclerosis

It is also important to remember that atherosclerosis starts at a young age. Research at a major institute found fatty streaks of atherosclerosis in the coronary arteries of boys as young as fifteen years of age. The risk factors are the same for teens and young professionals as for older people. People with the highest LDL cholesterol levels, the lowest HDL cholesterol levels, the highest blood pressures, and the highest blood-sugar levels have the most disease. And, of course, smoking and obesity increase the risk of atherosclerosis.

The Coronary Artery Risk Development in Young Adults (CARDIA) study found that young adults with certain risk factors were at greater risk of heart disease. Specifically, risk is

- three times greater for those with blood glucose greater than 110 mg/dl than those with lower levels;

- two times greater for those with an LDL above 130 mg/dl than those with lower levels;

- twice as high for those who smoked compared to those who did not smoke;

- one and a half times greater for those with blood pressure above 120/80 mm Hg than those with lower blood pressure; and

- one and a half times greater for those with a body mass index (BMI) over 25 kg/m^2 than more slender participants.

So remember, it's always a good idea to start taking care of your heart at an early age. You're never too young to take care of your blood-pumping muscle.

Important Points

- Heart disease is the number-one killer in the United States for *both* men and women. One out of every four American women dies of heart disease.

- Two types of heart disease, coronary MVD and broken heart syndrome, seem to affect more women than men.

- Both hormone replacement therapy and high-dosage birth control pills are risk factors for heart disease. And men don't take either.

- Young people, including athletes, are vulnerable to heart disease too.

- People often dismiss symptoms or risk factors in young people, especially among athletes.

- Hypertrophic cardiomyopathy affects one in every five hundred people, regardless of age.

CHAPTER 4

Taking Charge

YOU *CAN* MAKE A DIFFERENCE in your own life. According to the Centers for Disease Control and Prevention (CDC), there were more than 200,000 preventable deaths from heart disease and stroke in the United States in 2010. That's almost a quarter of a million deaths that didn't have to happen. You don't want you or your loved ones to fall into that category.

Research shows that living a healthy lifestyle can vastly improve your risk of heart disease. According to the American Heart Association, "Individuals can proactively lower their risk for cardiovascular disease and stroke by getting active, maintaining healthy blood pressure, cholesterol levels, weight and diet as well as avoiding smoking."

The American Heart Association also states, "Adopting healthier choices and effective preventative therapies can have an immediate effect on one's cardiovascular risk and help avoid becoming one of these preventable cardiovascular deaths."

Women with a healthy, low-risk lifestyle may have as much as a 92 percent lower risk of sudden cardiac death compared to women with a high-risk profile, according to leading medical research.

You're never too old to improve your lifestyle. A National Institutes of Health (NIH) study shows that even people ages seventy to ninety with a healthy lifestyle reduce their chances of dying from heart disease by nearly two-thirds.

In earlier chapters, we've seen something of the risk factors for heart disease, as well as the screening protocols that help identify problems early. That's useful. But probably the most useful information in this book is *what to do about it*.

Having information about your risk of heart disease and then burying your head in the sand won't help you prevent illness or counteract any of its damage. But there are some very useful steps you can take to protect your heart. The first step, though, is to decide that you want to take charge of your heart health. Step into the driver's seat of your life.

Don't Be Overwhelmed

Sometimes the task of changing your lifestyle can be overwhelming. Some people find that tackling one change at a time is the easiest approach. The basic steps to taking control of your heart health are as follows:

1. Deciding to take charge
2. Having regular screenings
3. Thinking positively
4. Stopping smoking and limiting alcohol consumption
5. Getting active
6. Watching your diet and weight
7. Getting enough sleep
8. Focusing on your emotions
9. Experiencing spirituality/meditation
10. Getting family and social support

Remember, just deciding to take control, deciding to do something about your heart health, is already an important first step.

Deciding to take charge of your health can be very empowering. You're no longer just sitting there, hoping your heart will get stronger and your quality of life will improve—you are taking action to make it happen.

To do this, though, you need to be willing to change, and you need to think positively about your ability to do so. And, of course, you'll need to develop an action plan.

Developing an Action Plan

The first step to developing an action plan is to figure out what it is that you need to work on. Take a look at your risk factors and the results of screening tests, and you can get a sense of how serious the problem is—and what to do about it.

Is lack of exercise an issue? Are you concerned about your blood pressure? Determine what steps you can take to improve your own individual heart health. If, for instance, you're not active enough, it's time to focus on fitness. If the bigger concern is the way you're fueling your body, concentrate on nutrition.

Willingness to Change

Studies show that people who are willing to change are more able to do so than people who are just getting a lot of pressure from their spouse, parents, children, or friends.

In addition, people who are prepared to make one change are also often able to make another at the same time or shortly afterward. An NIH study found, for instance, that people who are willing to quit smoking are also more likely to be willing to increase their physical activity.

The Transtheoretical Model of Change

One approach to helping people change their behavior is called the transtheoretical model of change, which has been used to develop ways to effectively promote health behavior changes. The five stages to this process are as follows:

1. **Precontemplation.** Here you're not actually planning to do anything yet. It's kind of like preengagement; you're thinking about thinking about it.
2. **Contemplation.** In this stage, you are assessing whether you want to change your behavior and doing cost-benefit analyses in your head. You're planning how you might go about, say, changing your diet or getting more exercise. Sometimes people get stuck in this stage for a while.
3. **Preparation.** At this point, you are intending to take action, usually in the coming month. You've developed a plan of action and taken some first steps, such as signing

up for a health education class, joining a gym, buying self-help books, or making an appointment with a counselor or therapist.

4. **Action**. Now you're getting started on the plan you've developed. You're watching your fat intake, heading to the gym, using the nicotine patch—whatever it is you've decided would be helpful to improve your heart health. Vigilance against relapse is key here.

5. **Maintenance**. In this stage, you're working hard to prevent relapse, but you're probably not initiating any new changes. The good news is that the more success you experience, the more confident you become that you can keep going. The lower your LDL and triglyceride levels fall, for instance, the more motivated you feel to continue to make the lifestyle changes that are literally improving your health.

The Power of Positive Thinking

Heart-disease patients with positive attitudes live longer, according to the American Heart Association. The organization also encourages people to exercise more, which also improves heart health. Specifically, researchers found that

- the most positive patients had a 42 percent less chance of dying from heart disease or any other reason; and
- positive mood cut risk of heart-related hospitalizations.

Positive thinking is powerful for everyone, regardless of age, gender, socioeconomic status, emotional health, social support, or overall functional ability when hospitalized.

"We know there is a relationship between depression and increased rates of mortality," says John C. Barefoot, PhD, a researcher at Duke University Medical Center. "These findings demonstrate the magnitude of the impact of patient expectations on the recovery process above and beyond depression and other psychological or social factors."

What is it that optimistic people do so well? Researchers at a major health care center say that optimistic people more effectively use coping techniques such as following their treatment plan. It may also be that negative thoughts lead to tension and stress, which hurts the body.

Cognitive Behavioral Therapy

The catch is how do you become more optimistic? Is it ever possible to change your attitude, to go from seeing the glass half empty to viewing it as half full? A therapeutic approach called cognitive behavioral therapy (CBT) has been found to help. It enables you to change the way you think in several ways. Using these techniques, you start to do the following:

- Notice irrational thoughts about yourself.
- Learn to stop these negative thoughts.
- Replace negative thoughts with more accurate ones.
- Discover how to relax mind and body, which can lower stress levels.
- Improve your time management, which can also lower stress levels.

CBT can happen in one-on-one sessions with a therapist or in group sessions. How does it work? It is a goal-oriented process that focuses on two tasks:

- Cognitive restructuring, which involves changing thinking patterns
- Behavioral activation, which focuses on putting these thoughts into action to overcome obstacles

Remember, you are not "stuck" with the level of heart health you have today. With planning, assistance, and effort, you can develop a plan to improve your overall well-being, and then make that plan happen.

Important Points

- You can make a change in your risk of heart disease.
- You can strengthen your heart.
- A positive attitude helps improve heart disease.
- Cognitive behavioral therapy might help with developing a positive attitude.
- Being willing to change is key to making lifestyle improvements.
- Using the transtheoretical model of change is a way to make lifestyle improvements.

CHAPTER 5

Cardiovascular Disease
Screening and Early Detection

EVEN THOUGH PREVENTION AND EARLY detection are known to be very important in all kinds of medical diseases, when it comes to cardiovascular disease, both of these make the difference between life and death—the reason being that cardiovascular disease hits very quickly, and often very lethally, without warning. By the time we know that we have cardiovascular disease, it is already too late. The medical data tells us that 50 percent of those who develop a heart attack or stroke are unsuspecting, with no symptoms or known prior disease. Who can reverse the effect of a heart attack or a stroke (that is, if the patient survives the initial episode)? And even without reaching a catastrophic event like a stroke or a heart attack, who can repair a heart muscle that is damaged and dilated because of prolonged decrease in blood flow to the heart muscle or poorly controlled high blood pressure?

We talked about risk factors and risk stratification in a prior chapter. Based on your risk category, your doctor will order one of several noninvasive tests to guide your medical therapy, initiate more testing, and monitor your response to the risk reduction and reversal measures he or she has utilized to treat you.

Some major cardiovascular organizations differ in the way they endorse different tests as standard screening measures. It is important and beneficial to use any screening tests under your medical doctor's supervision and to follow up with the results afterward.

The best way to figure out your risk of heart disease is by having your doctor screen you on a regular basis, usually at your annual checkup. Once you know your risk level, you can make lifestyle changes that can cut your risk of heart disease, and maybe even repair damage if you've already had heart problems.

At this appointment, your doctor will likely screen for any heart issues. The most common screening tests recommended by the American Heart Association are as follows:

- Blood work (fasting lipoprotein profile, C-reactive protein, homocysteine, blood-glucose level)
- Blood pressure
- Body weight/BMI
- Carotid intimal medial thickness (IMT)
- Stress testing
- Echocardiogram

Not all doctors perform all of these tests routinely on every patient, but it's helpful to know about them. Let's take a look at each of these screening tests.

Fasting Lipoprotein Profile

The fasting lipoprotein profile is a blood test that measures your total cholesterol level as well as the components parts: LDL, HDL, and triglycerides. You do the blood test after a nine-to twelve-hour fast. The American Heart Association recommends having a fasting lipoprotein profile done every four to six years, starting at age twenty, unless, of course, you are at increased risk for heart disease, in which case your doctor might want to perform the test more often.

As mentioned earlier, cholesterol is a waxy, fatlike substance that occurs naturally in the body. Your body needs a certain amount to function properly, but if there's too much, it can combine with other substances in the blood to form plaque. The plaque will then stick to your arteries, narrowing them and slowing or even blocking blood flow to the body parts that need it.

Total cholesterol. Total cholesterol consists of HDL plus LDL:

- Less than 200 mg/dl is ideal.

+ 200 mm to 239 mg/dl is borderline high.
+ More than 240 mg/dl is high.

HDL (often called "good" cholesterol). HDL protects against heart disease. Higher numbers are better.
+ More than 60 mg/dl is ideal.
+ 41 mo 59 mg/dl is borderline.
+ Less than 40mg/dl is a major risk factor.

LDL ("bad" cholesterol) is the main source of cholesterol buildup and blockage in arteries. Here it's best to have a lower number:
+ Less than 100 mg/dl is ideal.
+ 100 m to 129 mg/dl is near optimal/above optimal.
+ 130 mto 159 mg/dl is borderline high.
+ 160 m to 189 mg/dl is high.
+ More than 190 mg/dl is very high.

Triglycerides. These are another form of fat in the blood. Less is better with triglycerides. If your triglyceride level is high, doctors usually treat it.
+ Less than 149 mg/dl is ideal.
+ 150 mm Hg to 199 mg/dl is borderline high.
+ More than 200 mg/dl is high.

C-Reactive Protein (CRP) Levels

While we know that high cholesterol causes heart disease, only about half the people who have heart attacks have high cholesterol, according to leading medical research. That discrepancy makes it harder to predict a person's risk, so doctors and researchers have been looking for another way to pinpoint the people truly at risk for heart disease. Although this research is still relatively recent, measuring levels of CRP is looking to be a useful approach.

C-reactive protein is produced by the liver, usually in response to some sort of inflammation somewhere in the body. Healthy people have only very small amounts of CRP in their bloodstream;

once there's an injury of some sort, such as heart disease, the liver starts churning out extra CRP to help repair the damage.

Studies have found that as the CRP level rises, so does the risk of having—or dying from—a heart attack, stroke, or other cardiovascular problems. But there is some question about whether this test is helpful for routine heart-health screening.

The American Heart Association recommends physicians perform a blood test to measure CRP levels only to confirm that a heart attack has taken place and to assess future risk of coronary heart disease.

Homocysteine

Homocysteine is an amino acid typically found in the blood. Studies have shown that high levels are related to a higher risk of several types of heart disease. Studies show that women's homocysteine levels tend to rise after menopause. Studies also show that homocysteine might be connected with atherosclerosis and damaged arteries, but according to the American Heart Association, there has been no causal link between the two.

Some studies recommend taking folic acid and B vitamin supplements to help break down the homocysteine in the bloodstream. But the American Heart Association is careful; it doesn't recommend widespread use of folic acid and B vitamin supplements to reduce risk of heart disease and stroke. Instead, the American Heart Association advises eating a healthy, balanced diet with plenty of fruits and vegetables, whole grains, and fat-free or low-fat dairy products.

Blood-Glucose Level

Diabetes is a major risk factor for heart disease. If you have diabetes, you are twice as likely to have heart disease as someone with normal blood-glucose levels; this possibility could be even worse for women.

In fact, people with type 2 diabetes have the same risk of heart attack as people who have already had heart attacks. When combined with other conditions—especially having high blood pressure and being overweight—diabetes can cause harmful changes to the heart. These changes add to the risk of heart disease.

To find out if you have diabetes, doctors typically check blood-sugar levels at least every three years after you reach age forty-five. High blood-glucose (sugar) levels can lead to increased deposits of fatty materials inside your blood vessel walls. These deposits can slow or clog the blood flow, forcing the heart to work harder in order to pump the blood everywhere it needs to go, and can possibly lead to heart disease.

Normally, the body breaks food down into glucose. Your blood carries glucose through your body to provide energy to your cells. Your cells then use a hormone called insulin to turn the glucose into energy.

If your blood-glucose level is high, you are at greater risk of developing insulin resistance, prediabetes, and type 2 diabetes. If you have type 2 diabetes, it means that your body doesn't use insulin properly and responds by making more insulin. If you have type 1 diabetes, your body doesn't make enough insulin, which causes the blood-sugar level to rise. Both types are hard on the heart.

If your blood-sugar/blood-glucose level is

- less than 60 mg/dl, it is too low;
- 60 mg/dl to 120 mg/dl, it is ideal; and
- more than 120 mg/dl, it is too high (this is dangerous).

High blood-sugar levels may indicate inadequate levels of insulin. This can be caused by diabetes medication, overeating, lack of exercise, or other factors.

Low blood-sugar levels can be caused by taking too much insulin, skipping or postponing meals, over exercising, consuming excessive amounts of alcohol, or other factors. Neither situation is good for you.

If you have diabetes, you and your doctor will develop a treatment plan to help get it under control and improve your heart health at the same time.

Blood Pressure

You should have your blood pressure checked at least every two years starting at age twenty. Doctors and nurses check blood pressure using a blood pressure monitor cuff that wraps around your forearm. If your blood pressure is higher than it should be, or if you have other risk factors for heart disease, your doctor may want to check your blood pressure more often. In fact, some doctors take your blood pressure every time you walk into the office, even if you're just there to get a flu shot.

The reason many doctors check blood pressure so often is that this test is the only way to find out if your blood pressure is high. In general, there are usually no telltale symptoms of hypertension (high blood pressure). And you really want to keep tabs on your blood pressure because high blood pressure greatly increases your risk of heart disease.

Basically, blood pressure refers to the force of your blood pushing against the walls of your arteries. When your heart beats, it pumps blood into your arteries. Blood pressure is highest when your heart beats (this is called systolic pressure); between beats, when your heart is at rest, your blood pressure falls (this is called diastolic pressure).

A blood pressure reading includes both the systolic and diastolic pressure readings, usually the systolic number followed by the diastolic number. For instance, if your blood pressure is ideal, you would have a reading of 120/80 mm Hg. You might also hear someone say, "Blood pressure is one twenty over eighty."

When the systolic number is

- less than 120 mmHg, your blood pressure is normal;
- 120 mmHg to 139 mmHg, your blood pressure is called prehypertension;
- 140 mmHg to 159 mmHg, you have high blood pressure—stage 1; and
- more than 160 mmHg, you have high blood pressure—stage 2.

When the diastolic number is

- less than 80 mmHg, your blood pressure is normal;
- 80 mmHg to 89 mmHg, your blood pressure is called prehypertension;
- 90 mmHg to 99 mmHg, you have high blood pressure—stage 1; and
- more than 100 mmHg, you have high blood pressure—stage 2.

If your blood pressure reading indicates prehypertension, it means you are in danger of having high blood pressure and should take steps to prevent it. Discuss the steps for lowering your blood pressure with your doctor. If your blood pressure registers as high (stage 1 or 2), your doctor will help you figure out how to improve your blood pressure level and improve your heart health.

Body Weight/BMI

Obesity is a risk factor for heart disease. You can measure your risk by using the body mass index (BMI), which you calculate using your weight and height. The higher your BMI, the greater your chance of high blood pressure and heart disease:

+ Less than 18.5 is considered underweight.
+ 18.5–24.9 is normal.
+ 25.0–29.9 is overweight.
+ More than 30 is considered obese.

Body shape is also involved in heart-disease risk. If your excess weight is around your middle, it is more of a concern for heart health than if the excess weight is around your hips. Risk rises if your waist size is greater than thirty-five inches for women and greater than forty inches for men.

The good news is that even a small weight loss—even just 5 percent to 10 percent of your current weight—can help lower your risk of heart disease. Later chapters in this work provide some approaches to addressing the dangers of being overweight, focusing on exercise and nutrition and weight control.

Electrocardiogram (EKG)

This very old, simple, noninvasive test can give us a great deal of information about cardiac conditions, including the following:

+ If the person had a prior heart attack
+ If the person is currently having a blockage in the heart
+ If the electric rhythm of the heart is disturbed
+ If the electric conduction system of the heart is now working properly

- If the muscles of the heart are thickened out of proportion to the person's age and body size.

Carotid Intimal Medial Thickness (IMT)

Measuring the thickness of the inner layers of the carotid artery gives doctors a good sense of your risk of heart disease, especially atherosclerosis. Genetics and environmental factors, such as diet, exercise, and cigarette smoke, combine to cause inflammation of these layers in addition to plaque buildup.

By using ultrasound technology to measure the inner layers of the carotid artery, doctors can actually quantify the amount of disease that is there. They can then use that information to predict your risk of various types of heart disease. Studies show that the method is quick and cost effective. And it works just as well for women as for men, young and old. This test, however, is generally not a standard part of the routine physical.

Cardiac Stress Testing

If your doctor has ever had you walk or run on a treadmill or pedal a stationary bike while monitoring your heart, you've had a stress test. Stress testing allows doctors to see how your heart works during physical stress. Often, people show no sign of heart disease when they're just sitting in a chair or lying on an examination table. But when you exercise, your heart has to work harder to keep up, and it needs more blood and more oxygen to do this. As a result, if your arteries are narrow, it is more likely to show up during a stress test.

Different modalities of stress tests were developed to increase accuracy and deal with different scenarios. They include the following:

- Exercise stress EKG
- Exercise stress nuclear test
- Exercise stress echocardiogram
- Chemical nuclear stress test
- Dobutamine echocardiogram stress test

Echocardiogram

This test uses ultrasound to take pictures of your heart. To perform the test, a technician waves a probe called a transducer over your chest. The probe creates sound waves that bounce off your heart and "echo" back to the probe. These sound waves show up as pictures on a digital monitor that the cardiologist can then "read" and use to diagnose any problems. The test, which is completely safe and has no side effects, allows doctors to see the following:

- Size and shape of your heart
- Size, thickness, and movement of your heart's walls
- How your heart moves
- Heart's pumping strength
- Functioning of the heart's valves
- Any blood leaking backward through your heart valves
- Thickness of the heart valves
- Any blood clots, tumors, or infectious growth
- Outer lining of the heart
- Functioning of the large blood vessels that enter and leave the heart
- Abnormal holes between the chambers of the heart

Typically, this is a follow-up test if earlier screenings indicate something concerning. However, some doctors conduct echocardiograms routinely at annual physical exams.

Coronary Calcium Scoring

A coronary calcium scan looks for specks of calcium (called calcifications) in the walls of the coronary arteries. Calcifications are an early sign of coronary heart disease (CHD). The test can show whether you're at increased risk for a heart attack or other heart problems before other signs and symptoms occur.

Two techniques can show calcium in the coronary arteries—electron beam computed tomography (EBCT) and multidetector computed tomography (MDCT). Both use an X-ray machine to make detailed pictures of the heart. Specialists then study the pictures to see whether you're at risk for heart problems in the next two to ten years.

Ankle-Brachial Index

The association between peripheral vascular disease (PVD) and coronary artery disease (CAD) is very high. Up to 70 percent of people with PVD have CAD as well.

Ankle-brachial index (ABI) is often used to diagnose PVD. The ABI compares blood pressure in your ankle to blood pressure in your arm. This test shows how well blood is flowing in your limbs and whether PVD is affecting your limbs.

A normal ABI result is 1.0 or greater (with a range of 0.90 to 1.30). The test takes about ten to fifteen minutes to measure both arms and both ankles. It may be done yearly to see whether PVD is getting worse.

Conclusion

NONINVASIVE CARDIAC TESTS PROVIDE IMPORTANT information about how healthy your heart is and where the problem spots might lie. But a screening test by itself won't improve your heart health. If any of these tests suggests that your heart isn't in top shape, you should take further steps, under the guidance of your doctor, to improve your heart, which will both lengthen and improve your life.

Top Heart-Health Screening Tests

1. Fasting lipoprotein profile (cholesterol and triglycerides)
2. C-reactive protein
3. Homocysteine
4. Blood-glucose level
5. Blood pressure
6. Body weight/BMI
7. Carotid IMT

8. Stress testing
9. Echocardiogram
10. Coronary calcium scoring
11. Ankle-brachial index

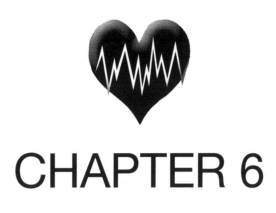

CHAPTER 6

Physical Activity

EVERYBODY KNOWS THAT EXERCISE HELPS you maintain a healthy body weight; increases your energy; builds up your abs, quads, and other muscles; and lowers your stress level. But did you know that exercise also lowers the risk of breast and colon cancer, boosts your mood and self-esteem while decreasing depression, improves the quality of your sleep, and cuts your risk of Alzheimer's disease? Exercise also prevents bone loss, helps you quit smoking, strengthens your immune system, and helps your body manage blood-sugar and insulin levels, lowering your risk for type 2 diabetes. It can delay or prevent chronic illnesses and diseases associated with aging, and as you get older, exercise helps you maintain your independence and quality of life. It can also be fun to hike with friends or take a family ski trip. Regular exercise can even improve your sex life.

Exercise even helps your emotional health. It increases the flow of oxygen, which directly affects the brain. Increased oxygen flow can improve your mental acuity and memory and relieve tension, anxiety, depression, and anger. At the same time, it promotes enthusiasm and optimism and enhances self-image.

Above all—at least for our immediate purposes—exercise is vital for heart health. Regular physical activity can help your heart in the following ways:

- Strengthening your heart muscle, thereby improving your heart's ability to pump blood to the lungs and throughout the body. As a result, more blood flows to your muscles and the oxygen levels in your blood rise.

- Improving blood cholesterol levels.
- Widening your capillaries, the body's tiny blood vessels. This allows them to deliver more blood throughout the body and take away more waste products.
- Lowering the risk of coronary heart disease.
- Lowering blood pressure and triglyceride levels.
- Raising your level of HDL cholesterol, the "good" cholesterol.
- Reducing levels of C-reactive protein, which is a sign of inflammation and is related to heart-disease risk.
- Lowering the risk of stroke by 20 percent to 27 percent.
- Decreasing risk of another heart attack among people who have had one already.

How Much Exercise Is Enough?

If you think you could be getting more exercise, there's a good chance you're right. For overall heart health, leading medical research recommends a combination of muscle strengthening and moderate or vigorous aerobic activity. But what's the difference between the two? It depends on the person; a professional basketball player and a librarian, for instance, might have different ideas of what constitutes moderate exercise.

In general, moderate exercise feels like a bit of a challenge. You can tell you're exercising moderately if

- your breathing quickens, but you're not out of breath;
- you develop a light sweat after about ten minutes; and
- you can carry on a conversation, but you can't sing.

Some common examples of moderate exercise include the following:

- Walking briskly (three miles an hour or faster, but not race walking)
- Water aerobics
- Bicycling slower than ten miles an hour
- Playing tennis (doubles)

+ Ballroom dancing
+ General gardening

Vigorous exercise involves a little more exertion. Again, it varies by person, but you can tell you're exercising vigorously if:

+ You are breathing deeply and rapidly.
+ You develop a sweat after only a few minutes.
+ You can't say more than a few words without pausing for breath.

Examples of vigorous exercise include the following:

+ Race walking, jogging, or running
+ Swimming laps
+ Playing tennis (singles)
+ Aerobic dancing or Zumba
+ Bicycling ten miles an hour or faster
+ Jumping rope
+ Heavy gardening (continuous digging or hoeing)
+ Hiking uphill or with a heavy backpack

Leading medical research recommends everyone get one of these three levels of activity every week:

+ At least thirty minutes of moderate-intensity aerobic activity at least five days a week for a total of 150 minutes a week, or
+ At least twenty-five minutes of vigorous aerobic activity at least three days a week for a total of seventy-five minutes, or
+ A combination of moderate- and vigorous-intensity aerobic activity

For additional health benefits, the American Heart Association recommends doing moderate- to high-intensity muscle-strengthening activity at least two days a week. If your goal is specifically to lower your blood pressure and cholesterol level, you should get an average of forty minutes of moderate to vigorous aerobic activity three or four times a week.

Bear in mind that vigorous exercise may not be safe for people who have had coronary heart disease. Check with your doctor before beginning a new regimen.

Physical Activity vs. Exercise

Physical activity is basically any body movement that works your muscles and requires more energy than resting. It includes activities such as the following:

- Walking
- Painting walls
- Dancing
- Swimming
- Yoga
- Gardening

Exercise is physical activity that's planned and structured. Examples include the following:

- Lifting weights
- Taking a Pilates or Zumba class
- Playing on a sports team
- Practicing yoga

Setting Fitness Goals

Fitness is highly individual, and you have to design an approach that works best for you. Here are a couple of factors to consider.

How fit are you? Some people start an exercise routine with unrealistic expectations; you don't want to overdo it. If you haven't walked more than two blocks in years, you might not want to start out with a 20K run. Think about questions such as *How long does it take me to walk a mile?* And *How many push-ups can I do in one minute*

What activities do you enjoy? Research shows that people are more likely to stick with programs that they enjoy. If, for instance, you enjoy competition, you might consider joining a team sport. If you enjoy being with others, a class might be more fun than exercising in your basement. If you like moving to music, think about Zumba or a dance aerobics class.

How much time do you have available? If you have a hard time fitting in thirty minutes a day, try breaking your workout up into ten- or fifteen-minute increments. Short spurts of aerobic exercise can be just as useful.

Finding Your Target Heart Rate

The way to figure out if you're exercising enough—or too much—is by assessing your heart rate as you exercise. To figure out your target heart rate, though, you have to start by determining your resting heart rate.

Your resting heart rate is the number of times your heart beats in a minute while it's at rest. Try checking your pulse in the morning before you get out of bed. The average resting heart rate is sixty to eighty beats per minute, but it varies by age and fitness level. To take your pulse, press the tips of your index and middle fingers lightly over the blood vessels in your wrist on the thumb side. Count your pulse for ten seconds and then multiply by six to find your beats per minute. That's your resting heart rate.

You can calculate your maximum heart rate with this formula:

$$220 - \text{your age}$$

Doctors recommend that people exercise at between 80 percent and 90 percent of their maximum heart rate. For instance, if you are fifty years old, you would determine your maximum heart rate in this way:

$$220 - 50 = 170$$

So your maximum heart rate would be 170. To stay between 80 percent and 90 percent of this maximum rate, you would want to exercise at a heart rate between 136 and 153 beats per minute.

Tips for Success

When you think about starting an exercise routine, a number of barriers often pop up. Sometimes you lack the time, motivation, or energy to stick with a routine. You may not have the resources or equipment to pursue your favorite activity. Or you may have a rough time squeezing exercise in amid a hectic work or travel schedule or child- or elder-care responsibilities. The key to overcoming these barriers is to think them through and find a solution to each potential problem; being proactive is the name of the game.

For instance, if you don't have much time, you could monitor your weekly activities and try to locate a few thirty-minute slots that are available. If you have child-care responsibilities, perhaps you can combine the two and play a high-intensity game of tag with the kids or do some pull-ups at the playground. And as for a heavy travel schedule, some fitness facilities (like the YMCA) have relationships with reciprocal memberships with facilities in other locations. If you put your mind to it, you can probably come up with a solution for at least most of these types of obstacles.

Here are a few recommendations that can improve your chances of success:

- Pick a time and place that fits neatly into your schedule.
- Exercise at the same time every day so it becomes a pattern.
- Do something you enjoy. And remember, you don't have to do the same thing every day; sometimes it's more fun to change it up.
- Listen to your body. If you feel pain, shortness of breath, dizziness, or nausea, take a break.
- Don't be discouraged if you miss a day—or a week. Go back to your routine gradually and work up to your old pace.
- Keep a record of your progress, and celebrate when you achieve special milestones.
- Above all, be kind to yourself. You're doing this whole thing to take care of your body.
- Be proud of yourself for the effort.

Start by Walking

You don't need fancy equipment or personal trainers to exercise. You can always just go for a walk. It's often the simplest approach to exercise—and has the lowest dropout rate of any physical activity, according to the American Heart Association. All you need are supportive shoes and comfortable clothes, and you can take a stroll in the woods, along a city street, on a treadmill at the gym, or even at the local mall. Here are some walking tips:

+ Start with short walks and build your way up to longer treks.
+ Breathe deeply. If you can't catch your breath, slow down. Don't worry about speed.
+ Think about your posture. Lift your head, pull your tummy in, and relax those shoulders.
+ There's no reason to carry hand weights. They just put extra stress on your elbows and shoulders.
+ If you decide you want to pick up the pace, don't change your stride—just speed up your motions.
+ You can add challenge by climbing hills or by varying your tempo (one block slow, one block fast).

Start with a relaxed pace to warm up, and then gradually increase your speed. But you don't have to run if you don't want to; walking briskly can lower your risk of high blood pressure, high cholesterol, and diabetes as much as running, according to a major research institution. At the end of the walk, when you're all warmed up, you can stretch your hamstrings, calves, chest, shoulders, and back. That will help prevent muscle cramping the next day.

Important Points

+ Physical activity lowers the risk of heart disease.
+ It also offers many other benefits to your physical and mental health.
+ For maximum benefit, you should exercise most days of the week.
+ It helps to pick an activity that you enjoy and that fits easily into your lifestyle. You can always switch to a different activity.
+ Keep an eye on your heart rate as you exercise to make sure you don't do too little—or too much.
+ Walking is a great way to start incorporating exercise into your daily life.

CHAPTER 7

Nutrition/Weight Control

JUST LIKE YOU WOULDN'T POUR a glass of milk or orange juice into your gas tank and expect your car to run smoothly, you don't want to pour the wrong fuel into your body and hope it will all work out. You want to give your body the best possible fuel to keep it running as long and as well as possible.

Fueling your body with the right mix will provide you with vitality and energy, boost your immune system, enhance your ability to concentrate and improve your mood, help you stay at the right weight, and keep you active and fit. And, of course, it will contribute to your heart health.

Researchers working on the Framingham Nutrition Studies, which focused specifically on women, found that those who consumed a heart-healthy diet and had never smoked cut their risk for subclinical heart disease by more than 80 percent, compared to smokers with less heart-healthy diets. The catch is that it can be difficult to change your diet. After all, you've been eating a certain way, falling into certain patterns, for years. But remember: every change is important—and it's the overall pattern of choices that counts. If you mess up on a snack one afternoon, don't give up. Just use it as a reminder to be more mindful of what you eat the next time you sit down at the table.

Consider these guidelines when planning your meals:

- Eat more fruits and vegetables. Aim for four or five servings each of fruits and vegetables every day. That includes 100 percent vegetable or fruit juice. Fruits and veggies are low in saturated fat and cholesterol and high in fiber. In general, try to fill at least half your plate with colorful vegetables.

+ Eat more whole-grain foods. These include whole-wheat bread, rye bread, brown rice, and whole-grain cereal.

+ Use liquid vegetable oils, such as olive, canola, corn, or safflower, to cook with instead of solid fats like butter or Crisco. While you're at it, limit how much fat or oil you use in order to lower the amount of trans fat you consume.

+ Select fat-free, 1 percent fat, and low-fat dairy products.

+ Opt for chicken, fish, and beans rather than beef, pork, and lamb. In general, skinless poultry, fish, and vegetable protein (like beans and tofu) are lower in saturated fat and cholesterol than other meats. Eating oily fish containing omega-3 fatty acids (think salmon, trout, and herring) can help lower your risk of death from heart disease.

+ Watch your sodium intake. Aim to eat no more than 2,400 mg of sodium a day. If you can, it would be even better to reduce your daily intake to 1,500 mg. And remember, both soy sauce and teriyaki sauce have lots of sodium.

+ Be careful about saturated fat; aim for saturated fats to encompass no more than 5 percent to 6 percent of your total calories consumed. With a diet of 2,000 calories a day, that's about thirteen grams of saturated fat.

+ Watch out for foods and drinks with added sugar. Just because it says it's an energy drink doesn't mean it's good for you.

+ Limit your alcohol consumption, and avoid smoking and secondhand smoke.

When you prepare food at home, you know what's in it and how it was cooked. That's probably the best way to watch your nutrition. Also, try to avoid prepared foods; they are usually loaded with sodium. You have more control over what you eat when you control how you make it.

Keep an eye on portion size. You don't want to take in more calories than you expend. And if you want to lose weight, you'll need to lower your calorie intake and increase your physical activity even more.

One research study found that middle-aged people who gained between eleven and twenty-two pounds after age twenty substantially increased their risk of developing heart disease and high blood pressure, among other conditions. Specifically, the risk tripled with excess weight gain. Those who gained more than twenty-two pounds had an even higher increased risk.[1]

Calculating Calorie Requirements

To figure out how many calories you should consume each day, start with your current weight and multiply it by fifteen. That's how many calories you need to eat every day to maintain your body weight, if you are moderately active. Moderate activity means exercising at least thirty minutes a day by doing activities like walking briskly, climbing stairs, or active gardening. (There are also multiple calculators on different websites that will do the calorie calculations for you.)

To lose weight, you need to eat less.

For instance, if you're a forty-five-year-old woman who is five feet five and weighs 145 pounds and you live an active lifestyle, you need to eat 2,000 calories a day to maintain your weight.

So, if you want to lose a pound or two a week—a rate that experts consider safe—you should eat 500 to 1,000 calories less than what you need to maintain your weight.

Losing How-To

Here are some recommendations for how to maintain a weight-loss diet:

- Keep your portions smaller than your fist. Smaller portions make it easier to eat less. It can also help to use smaller dishes; if the plate looks full, you might be more satisfied.
- Fill up on low-calorie foods. Soups, salads, fruits, and vegetables can help you feel full while adding fewer calories than, say, grabbing a cookie or candy bar.
- Keep a food diary. If you write down what you eat every day, it's easier to keep track of what you're eating.
- If you want to indulge in a favorite food, try doing a trade-off. Eat a lower-calorie meal and then take a small bite of dessert. Also, try having dessert after lunch instead of after dinner; that gives you more time to burn off those calories.

---

[1] E. B. Rimm et al., "Body size and fat distribution as predictors of coronary heart disease among middle-aged and older US men," *American Journal of Epidemiology* 141, no. 12 (1995):1117–27.

+ Try eating more frequent, yet smaller meals. If you have a little something every three or four hours, you're less apt to feel hungry. Just make sure to track those calories; if you eat more meals of the same size, you'll defeat your purpose.

+ Don't shop for groceries when you're hungry. It's just asking for trouble. If you really can't time it right, at least stop and have a quick and healthy snack before you grab that shopping cart.

+ Increase exercise. The more calories you burn, the fewer that stay on your body. The key is to eat a little less and move a little more.

The Effect of a Healthy Diet on the Brain

A healthy diet and regular exercise can also protect the brain and ward off mental disorders. Some particularly useful foods include the following.

Omega-3 fatty acids. Found in salmon, walnuts, and kiwi, omega-3 can improve your learning and memory and protect against depression and mood disorders, bipolar disorder, schizophrenia, and dementia.

Folic acid. Present in spinach, orange juice, and yeast, folic acid is essential to brain function. It can prevent against cognitive decline and dementia and enhance the effect of antidepressants. (Pregnant women often take a folic acid supplement to prevent birth defects of the brain and spinal cord.)

Vitamin E. Nuts and seeds are a good source of vitamin E, which can protect against cognitive decline.

Antioxidants. Found in many vegetables (e.g., kale, spinach, brussels sprouts, alfalfa sprouts, broccoli, beets, red bell pepper, onion, corn, eggplant) and fruits (e.g., prunes, raisins, blueberries, blackberries, strawberries, raspberries, plums, oranges, red grapes, cherries), antioxidants reduce the risk of heart disease and stroke and protect brain cells.

Sodium. You have to be careful about sodium, also known as sodium chloride. A certain amount of it is essential for the body to function properly. But too much sodium can pull water into your arteries and veins, increasing blood pressure. Over time, this increased pressure can overstretch or injure the blood vessels and build up plaque, which can block blood flow. The American Heart Association recommends getting about 1,500 mg of sodium a day;

unfortunately, most Americans consume more than twice that much (more along the lines of 3,400 mg daily).

To cut your sodium consumption, try avoiding these six saltiest foods:

+ Breads and rolls
+ Cold cuts and cured meats
+ Pizza
+ Poultry
+ Soup
+ Sandwiches

Watching sodium consumption is most important among certain populations. Eating too much sodium has the strongest effect on African Americans; people over age fifty; and anyone with high blood pressure, diabetes, or kidney disease.

Preparation at Home

Cooking your own food is probably the best way to guarantee that you know what went into your food and how it was prepared. Plus, you can save money at the same time.

Often, people plan their meals out for the week. Use heart-healthy recipes with lean meats, whole grains, and plenty of vegetables and fruits. It helps to always have extra-virgin olive oil in a spray bottle (you use less than when you pour it), an egg substitute, and fat-free or light soymilk on hand.

Be careful when you pick your meats. "Choice" and "select" beef generally has less fat than "prime." Also, "loin" and "round" cuts have less fat. When you're eating chicken, stick to the white meat instead of the fattier dark meat. Be sure to remove the skin of the chicken; that's the worst culprit in terms of fat.

Think about how you prepare foods. Try to avoid frying, which creates food high in fat and calories. Instead, bake, broil, or sauté chicken, and grill, broil, or poach fish. You can even dice and microwave onions with a little bit of water instead of frying them.

It's better to use vegetable oils or nonfat cooking sprays for cooking rather than solid oils. Try to stick with canola oil, corn oil, olive oil, safflower oil, sesame oil, soybean oil, and sunflower oil, which are among the lowest in saturated fats, trans fats, and cholesterol. But use them sparingly, as they are still high in calories. Try to avoid coconut, palm, and palm kernel oils.

When it comes to adding a little spice to your life—or at least to your cooking—beware of salt. It doesn't just come in the container marked "salt." Packaged seasoning mixes often contain a lot of sodium, which is not ideal. It's better to use fresh herbs and grind them with a mortar and pestle for the most flavor.

There are lots of options you may not use regularly. Vinegar and citrus juice enhance flavors, and hot peppers will definitely spice up your meal.

Eating Out

All of the previous advice is great when you know exactly what goes into your food and how it was prepared. Eating out, though, brings up another set of issues.

Picking a Restaurant

Lots of restaurants offer dishes that are low in saturated fats, trans fats, and cholesterol. Some places will even make your food to order, especially if you're a regular. When you pick a restaurant, keep in mind these two tips:

+ Avoid all-you-can-eat buffets; along with all that food, they're offering unlimited temptation to eat too much or to eat the wrong things.
+ If you know the restaurant, decide what you want to order in advance; that way you're less apt to be tempted by a less healthy option.

Ordering a Meal

If you order carefully, you can eat out as healthily as you can at home. Start by doing the following:

+ Look for dishes marked "healthy."
+ Talk to your server if you're unsure. Ask about the ingredients and how the dish is prepared. You can also ask which dishes are the healthiest options.

+ Ask for healthy substitutions: see if you can have a baked potato instead of French fries, vegetables rather than onion rings, or a salad instead of coleslaw.

To avoid fat and calories, steer clear of foods that are:

+ Fried or pan-fried
+ Au gratin
+ Crispy
+ Scalloped
+ Sautéed
+ Buttered
+ Creamed
+ Stuffed

Instead, choose foods that are:

+ Steamed
+ Broiled
+ Baked
+ Grilled
+ Poached
+ Roasted

Other considerations:

+ Don't order entrées with fatty meats.
+ Pick seafood, chicken, or lean meat.
+ Be careful with cocktails, appetizers, and bread and butter—extra fat, sodium, and calories can sneak up on you, even in small portions. (And just because it comes free with the meal doesn't mean it doesn't contain calories, fat, and sodium.)
+ Ask for butter, cream cheese, salad dressing, sauce, and gravy on the side so you can decide exactly how much to use. And use these as sparingly as you can; it defeats the purpose if you dump the entire side order onto your meal.

- Ask for your food to be prepared with monosaturated oils (olive, canola, and peanut oils) and polysaturated oils (soybean, corn, safflower, and sunflower oils).

Salad-Bar Pointers

- Pick fresh greens, raw vegetables, fresh fruits, and garbanzo beans. Opt for reduced-fat, low-fat, light, or fat-free dressings.
- Stay away from cheeses, marinated salads, pasta salads, and fruit salads with whipped cream.
- Be sparing with nuts; they are a good source of protein, but they also contain plenty of calories.

Fast Food

When you hear "fast food," you probably think unhealthy. But these days, most fast-food chains offer a few good options. You just have to order carefully and avoid supersizing. Whenever possible, opt for the following:

- Grilled chicken
- Salads (without high-fat dressings)
- Low-fat milk
- Fruit
- Oatmeal

Remember, watching what you eat can have a real effect on your heart health. A healthy lifestyle, which includes eating well and exercising regularly, can reduce your risk of heart disease by as much as 80 percent, according to leading medical research.

Important Points

Nutrition can have a huge effect on physical health—and especially on the heart.

- Eat more healthy foods.

- Eat less of the foods that aren't as good for you.
- Try to avoid prepared foods.
- When you cook, think about the foods you use and how you prepare them. Avoid frying.
- Get plenty of exercise; balancing what you eat with what you do can help you maintain a healthy weight.
- You can eat out—just keep a careful eye on the menu.

CHAPTER 8

Healthy Sleep

SLEEP ISN'T JUST WHAT HAPPENS during those hours when you're not awake. Your body is actually very busy while you're sleeping, and when you wake up, you reap the benefits.

Getting enough sleep—and getting good-quality sleep—makes it easier to learn and focus your attention. It decreases the risk of obesity, improves your blood-sugar level (which decreases the risk of diabetes), boosts your immune system, and triggers the body to release the hormones that promote normal growth and help repair cells and tissues.

Most important—at least for us right now—sleep is good for your heart. Deep sleep helps your body heal and repairs your heart and blood vessels. If you don't get enough sleep over a long period of time, you're at increased risk for heart disease, high blood pressure, and stroke, among other health problems.

Specifically, if you don't get enough sleep, your body releases more adrenaline, cortisol, and other hormones, which keep your blood pressure from dropping at night, and this increases your risk of heart disease. Not getting enough sleep can also trigger your body to produce more of certain proteins that may well play a role in heart disease. For instance, people who don't get enough sleep often have high levels of C-reactive protein, a sign of increased risk of atherosclerosis or hardening of the arteries.

How Much Sleep Is Enough?

The amount of sleep needed varies person to person and even over the course of one's lifetime. Basically, you need less sleep as you go along. The National Lung, Heart, and Blood Institute recommends the following number of hours of sleep every day:

Newborns	*16–18 hours*
Preschool-aged children	*11–12 hours*
School-aged children	*At least 10 hours*
Teens	*9–10 hours*
Adults (including the elderly)	*7–8 hours*

If you regularly sleep less than the recommended number of hours, the loss adds up. An adult who sleeps five hours a night, for instance, racks up a sleep deficit of fourteen hours in a single week. And over a month, or several months, well, it really adds up.

Sleep deprivation isn't good for anyone, but it is apparently harder on women than men. A study at a major medical center found that women who sleep less than six hours a night had far more inflammation than men who slept the same amount.

Some people try to catch up on their sleep deficit by taking naps or sleeping more on weekends or days off. But neither approach is as good as getting the amount of sleep needed every night. Naps give a short boost of energy, but don't provide all the benefits of deep sleep. And sleeping different amounts every day upsets your sleep-wake rhythm.

You can tell you're not getting enough sleep if you're ready to doze off while doing one of the following:

+ Reading or watching TV
+ Sitting still in a public place, such as a movie theater, meeting, or classroom
+ Riding in a car for an hour without stopping
+ Relaxing and talking to someone
+ Sitting quietly after a meal
+ Waiting in traffic for a few minutes

What Is Good-Quality Sleep?

There are two types of sleep: rapid eye movement (REM) sleep and non-REM sleep. You start out in non-REM sleep, which consists of three stages:

Stage 1: You're sleeping lightly and are easily awakened. Your muscles relax, and your heart and breathing rates begin to slow.

Stage 2: Brain waves slow down, with occasional bursts of rapid waves. You spend about half the night in this stage.

Stage 3: Brain waves get even slower, with few rapid waves. It's hard to be awakened. Bedwetting and sleepwalking tend to happen in this stage.

People usually enter REM sleep after about sixty to ninety minutes of sleep. This phase is even deeper than stage 3 non-REM sleep. Your eyes move rapidly in different directions, though your eyelids stay closed. Breathing becomes more rapid, irregular, and shallow, and your heart rate and blood pressure increase. You cannot move your arm or leg muscles. People usually dream during REM sleep.

You go through the sleep stages throughout the night. Each complete cycle takes about ninety minutes. Both REM and non-REM stages are important for heart health. Researchers figure you need four or five full sleep cycles to get "a good night's sleep."

The more interrupted your sleep, the worse your night's sleep.

Sleep Disorders

Sometimes people experience a sleep disorder that keeps them from getting their enough hours of sleep per night. The most common kinds are sleep disorders are as follows:

- *Insomnia*: Having a hard time falling or staying asleep
- *Sleep Apnea*: Breathing interruptions of at least ten seconds during sleep
- *Restless Legs Syndrome*: A tingling or prickly sensation in the legs

- *Narcolepsy*: Daytime "sleep attacks"
- *Parasomnias*: Includes nightmares, night terrors, sleepwalking, sleep talking, head banging, wetting the bed, and grinding your teeth

Sleep Apnea

Despite its name, this is actually a sleep-related breathing disorder. There are two types of sleep apnea:

- **Obstructive Sleep Apnea**: This is the more common type of sleep apnea that happens when the muscles at the back of the throat don't keep the airways open.
- **Central Sleep Apnea**: This type of sleep apnea occurs when the brain doesn't properly control breathing during sleep.

Aside from the obvious—not getting enough sleep—there are several other signs of sleep apnea. These include the following:

- Snoring
- Difficulty concentrating
- Depression
- Irritability
- Sexual dysfunction
- Learning and memory difficulties
- Falling asleep while at work, on the phone, or while driving

Probably the most effective way to treat sleep apnea is by using a continuous positive airway pressure (CPAP) device. This is a mask that fits over the nose or mouth and gently blows air into the airway to help keep it open during sleep. It looks a little odd, but it is pretty effective at helping you to do the following:

- Lose weight
- Avoid alcohol
- Quit smoking

How to Improve Your Sleep

There are a couple of key ways to improve the quality of your sleep. These include the following:

+ Stick to a regular sleep schedule—go to bed and wake up at the same time every day, weekends and weekdays.
+ Spend some time outside every day, and if you can, be physically active.
+ Avoid caffeine and nicotine. Caffeine can stay in your body for up to eight hours.
+ Avoid alcoholic drinks before bed.
+ Avoid large meals and beverages late at night; a light snack, however, is OK.
+ Don't nap after 3:00 p.m.
+ Use the hour before bed to get ready. Avoid strenuous exercise and bright light, which tell the body that it's time to be awake. Instead, try to take it easy—maybe read a book, take a hot bath, or use other relaxation techniques.
+ Keep your bedroom quiet, cool, and dark; a dim nightlight is fine.

Important Points

+ Getting enough sleep is key.
+ Getting good-quality sleep is most useful.
+ All stages of sleep are important for heart health.
+ As we get older, we need less sleep, but people at every age need more sleep than they typically think.
+ There are concrete, nonmedicinal ways to improve the quantity and quality of your sleep.

CHAPTER 9

Emotional Issues

THE CONNECTION BETWEEN THE HEART as a muscle and the heart as a metaphor for our emotions is stronger than it seems. Your emotions, moods, and personality can affect the health of your blood-pumping heart.

Some of these emotional issues can cause atherosclerosis, the slow process of hardening of the arteries that puts you at risk for heart disease. Other issues can be the "last straw" that sets off a heart attack or stroke. Negative emotions can speed up the heartbeat, cause blood pressure to rise, and can even change the heart's electrical stability. And all of that can lead to heart disease.

This issue isn't one to ignore. Research shows that your emotional health can affect your heart health as much as smoking, high blood pressure, obesity, and cholesterol problems.

The biggest concerns include the following:

+ Depression
+ Anger/hostility
+ Anxiety
+ Social isolation
+ Stress

In addition, studies have shown that having a positive attitude can really help your heart health.

Experiencing a little bit of these emotions isn't a bad thing; in fact, it can be helpful in certain circumstances. If you're crossing the street and see a car coming, for instance, a little bit of anxiety might get you moving faster. Similarly, a little stress can get you to finish a project on a tight deadline. The key is to have these emotional responses help you, not hurt you.

Be Positive

Having a positive attitude toward life and optimism about your health can improve your health. Researchers suggest that these four qualities are particularly beneficial:

+ A sense of enthusiasm and hopefulness
+ A feeling that good things will happen—and that you can make them happen
+ Supportive networks of friends and family
+ Being able to bounce back from stressful times

People with positive attitudes may just take better care of themselves by exercising more, eating a more healthful diet, and being better about taking necessary medications. It's hard to know which came first: the healthy lifestyle or the positive attitude.

Researchers in the Netherlands found that heart patients with positive attitudes were more likely to exercise and had less chance of dying during a five-year follow-up study.[2]

But it's not always easy to change your approach from glass half empty to glass half full. It's not like your doctor will tell you to take two jokes and call him in the morning. Alas, it is a little bit more complicated.

Sometimes changing your approach is just a matter of what the American Heart Association calls "positive self-talk." Instead of saying to yourself, "I can't do this," try saying, "I'll do the best I can." Instead of thinking, "I'll never get healthy," try telling yourself, "I'm doing a little better every day."

It also helps to inject some giggles into your daily life. Watch a favorite movie or TV show, read a humorous novel or enjoy some cartoons (whatever makes you laugh), hang out with friends who don't hesitate to be silly, or play games with your kids. Whatever improves your mood—and your attitude—do it regularly.

---

[2] *Circulation: Cardiovascular Quality and Outcomes* 6 (2013): 559–566. doi: 10.1161/CIRCOUTCOMES.113.000158.

Depression

Feeling a little down, blue, or sad is normal. Earning a bad grade in a class, not getting an ideal job assignment, or having a fight with a good friend can leave you feeling a little dejected.

Depression, though, is a completely different experience. It interferes with daily life and makes it difficult to work, sleep, study, eat, and enjoy life. And it lasts a lot longer than a few hours or even a few days. A persistent depressive disorder, according to the National Institutes of Mental Health, can extend for more than two years. There are several kinds of depression, including psychotic depression, postpartum depression, and seasonal affective disorder.

For years, doctors and researchers have known that heart disease and depression are closely linked. People with heart disease are more likely to experience depression than people without heart disease. Angina and heart attacks are closely linked with depression.

For years, researchers thought that the connection between depression and heart health was behavioral. People with depression, they reasoned, are less likely to make the sorts of lifestyle changes that can improve heart health. They're less likely to exercise regularly, watch what they eat, and take heart medication on the proper schedule—and are more likely to smoke and drink.

At the same time, researchers figured that having heart disease in itself was a cause of depression. It's certainly not a cheerful thought to have such a worrisome disease; it can certainly put a damper on one's mood.

But recent research suggests a physiological connection between the two disorders. A recent study published in the *Journal of the American Heart Association* found that women at or below age fifty-five are twice as likely to suffer a heart attack or require artery-opening surgery if they are moderately or severely depressed. "Women in this age group are also more likely to have depression, so this may be one of the 'hidden' risk factors that can help explain why women die at a disproportionately higher rate than men after a heart attack," says study author Amit J. Shah, MD,

Specifically, the study found the following:

- Women at or below age fifty-five who were more depressed had a 7 percent increase in the presence of heart disease.
- In men and older women, symptoms of depression didn't predict the presence of heart disease.

- Women fifty-five and younger were 2.2 times as likely to suffer a heart attack, die of heart disease, or require an artery-opening procedure if they had moderate or severe depression.
- Women fifty-five and younger were 2.5 times as likely to die from any cause during the follow-up period if they had moderate or severe depression.

Another study by psychiatrists and cardiologists at the University of California at Davis and Duke University Schools of Medicine found that controlling depression in patients with heart failure can improve health status, social functioning, and quality of life.[3] In addition, patients with reduced depression could walk, on average, forty-seven meters—or about 154 feet—farther than their counterparts with major depression.

Improving depression through medication and talk therapy can improve overall health and decrease risk of heart disease.

Anger

Hotheads can sometimes pay the price in heart health. Explosive people who frequently hurl objects and scream at the top of their lungs are at greater risk of heart disease. In fact, people who are quick to anger are more likely to develop premature heart disease than calmer people and are five times more likely to have an early heart attack, according to leading medical research.

We're not talking about people who curse when they stub their toe; that includes most of us. If anything, being able to express reasonable anger is healthy because it keeps us from bottling these emotions inside ourselves. It's a question of degree.

Much like stress, emotions such as anger and hostility activate the "fight-or-flight" response, which speeds your heart rate, pumps adrenaline and cortisol into your system, and gives you a burst of energy.

And all of that extra activity causes your heart to pump harder, makes your blood vessels constrict, and damages your artery walls. Just as stress raises your blood pressure, so does extreme

[3] CIRCHEARTFAILURE.112.967620. Published online before print. October 12, 2012. doi: 10.1161/ CIRCHEARTFAILURE.112.967620.

anger. Leo Pozuelo, MD, section head of consultation psychiatry and staff at the Heart and Vascular Institute at the Cleveland Clinic, says that anger does the following:

- Raises cortisol levels
- Increases platelet reactivity
- Alters the natural autonomic tone that we have in the heart
- Increases inflammatory markers

The risk of a show of temper is minimal—about one extra heart attack for every 10,000 people each year—but the risk of heart attack increases as the incidents of anger rise. For instance, if you have five episodes of irritation a day, your chances of cardiovascular events rise by about 158 extra heart attacks per 10,000 people a year.

Anxiety

The effect of anxiety on heart health hasn't been studied as much as depression, but experts believe there is a connection between the twoGeneralized anxiety disorder (GAD), which is the term for having an excessive amount of anxiety on most days, can cause an increased risk of heart disease. Women are about twice as likely to experience anxiety as men.

When you're feeling anxious, it can affect your heart health in several ways:

- Increase your heart rate; sometimes it can even interfere with normal heart function and add to the risk of sudden cardiac arrest.
- Boost your blood pressure; high blood pressure can lead to coronary disease, weakening of the heart muscle, and heart failure.
- Decrease your heart rate variability; this is dangerous after an acute heart attack and can raise the risk of death.

Social Isolation

Everyone knows that we need to connect with others. Without connections, we don't function as well at our jobs, at school, or in our families.

But feeling lonely isn't the same as physically being alone. Lonely people are as likely as anyone else to be surrounded by coworkers, neighbors, friends, and family. Being lonely means feeling isolated, feeling that these relationships aren't enough somehow to meet your social needs. You can be surrounded by people and feel lonely or work and live alone, yet be perfectly happy with the situation.

Studies show that loneliness is connected to depression—and also to higher blood pressure, increased cortisol (a hormone released in response to stress), and less restful sleep.

We experience physical symptoms as well. People who feel socially isolated experience increased blood pressure, deteriorated immune systems, and less restful sleep. Some studies suggest that loneliness is as much of a risk factor for overall health as obesity and smoking.

Part of it has to do with "executive functioning." Some studies suggest that loneliness affects the ability to control your thoughts, emotions, and impulses. Lonely people are more likely to have more fat and sugar in their diets and less exercise in their daily lives than people who are happier; similarly, lonely people are prone to alcoholism and drug addiction.

People who are lonely tend to focus more on negative thoughts and perceptions than people who aren't feeling lonely. They tend to find greater fault with themselves and with those around them; they expect others to be less friendly, less kind. And this becomes a self-fulfilling prophecy—they experience what they expect to experience.

The reverse is true as well. People who get plenty of support from friends, family, and a larger community have a lower risk for heart disease than people who don't. And this is true even among people who have a lot of physical risk factors.

Stress

In prehistoric times, a stressful situation was very tangible; for instance, it might have been the real threat of being eaten by a saber-toothed tiger. So our bodies developed what we call a fight-or-flight response. Our body releases a number of chemicals, including cortisol and epinephrine (adrenaline), to prepare us for action.

The catch is that these days, a stressful situation is a different matter. Having a burst of adrenaline doesn't really help when what's causing the stress is, for instance, standing in line at the grocery store while the woman in front of you fights over a can of tuna fish.

Stress affects your heart in both direct and indirect ways. Directly, it can raise your blood pressure and change the way your blood clots, which can lead to a heart attack. It also affects other parts of your body; stress causes headaches and back, shoulder, and stomach pains. It can zap your energy; mess up your sleep patterns; and leave you feeling cranky, forgetful, and out of control. When stress continues, when you experience what we call chronic stress, your body stays on "high alert," off and on, for days or weeks. That's even harder on the body and weakens your immune system.

To cope with all of these symptoms, people sometimes drink, smoke, overeat, consume too much sodium, or stop exercising. Chronic stress can weaken the immune system and cause headaches and stomachaches. All of these behavioral changes are also bad for the body overall and increase the risk for heart disease.

Emotions and Heart Patients

The period after heart-disease diagnosis can be confusing, scary, and frightening and can lead to a period of emotional upset. In fact, after heart problems, up to 65 percent of coronary heart-disease patients experience some sort of depression, anxiety, isolation, or diminished self-esteem, according to the National Institutes of Mental Health (NIMH). And, of course, that can complicate the recuperation process and lead to worse outcomes.

Specifically, heart patients often feel one or more of the following:

+ Uncertain about the future
+ Concerned about the ability to be a productive employee, mother, father, daughter, son, and so on
+ Guilty about previous habits that might have increased their heart attack risk
+ Embarrassed and worried about diminished physical capabilities

Of course, if you're having these sorts of feelings, they will complicate your recuperation process. They can affect you physically, leading to changes in your nervous system and hormonal balances, which can then lead to heart rhythm disturbances. These feelings can also cause uncommonly sticky platelets, which can accelerate development of atherosclerosis (hardening of the arteries) and increase the risk of heart attack.

In addition, people with depression may have a more difficult time keeping up with healthy behaviors, such as the following:

- Taking heart medications properly
- Exercising
- Eating properly
- Stopping smoking
- Limiting alcohol consumption
- Holding a positive attitude about the future

All of these behaviors can combine to increase the risk of further heart disease.

It's important to recognize any of these feelings and figure out how to deal with them. Support groups, one-on-one therapy, and medication are some of the ways that people cope. Remember, if you deal with these negative feelings after heart problems, you are more likely to have a positive outcome.

Relieving Stress

There are as many ways to relieve stress as there are things that cause it in the first place—everything from suggestions that you only check your e-mail three times a day to advising that you eat a bit of chocolate to relax. The key is to figure out what works for you.

Here are some recommendations that might help:

- Take care of your body. This involves regular exercise, eating healthy, and getting enough sleep. Find time to relax every single day. If you're good to your body, it will be good to you.
- Avoid stressors. Learn to say no or to delegate responsibilities. Limit activities—or people—who cause you stress. If you feel less stress, you'll have less to work on.
- Pamper yourself. Whether that means getting a foot massage or going to a sauna, indulging in a chocolate-covered strawberry, or taking a bubble bath, give it a try on a regular basis. (Well, watch it with the chocolate treats.) You're worth it.

+ Spend quality time with others. Consider hanging out with friends, meeting new people, volunteering in your community, or seeking counseling. Make those human connections that bring joy to your life.

+ Have quality time alone. You can keep a journal, meditate, take a walk in nature, or try yoga. Feel comfortable being by yourself.

+ Cram more fun into your life. Find a hobby you enjoy—anything from listening to music to gardening, from sketching to flying kites. Laugh more; laughing can be a good way to guarantee a good number of belly laughs. Exercise those smile muscles. It's good for you.

Deal with Depression and Anxiety

The first thing to remember is that depression and anxiety are perfectly normal conditions, not character flaws. It's not your fault you feel depressed or anxious. Understanding that is the first step toward alleviating the symptoms.

The second step is asking for help, which is not always easy. You can confide in someone you trust, like a friend, family member, or member of the clergy. They can offer a sympathetic ear, which may just do the trick.

Consider talking to a health care professional. They can offer professional counseling, medication, or a combination of the two. Remember, there are different types of talk therapy, as well as different medications. You and your doctor have to figure out what is best for you and your situation.

Also, remember that taking care of your body is important. People experiencing depression or anxiety may be so focused on their mental state that they forget this, but it can help enormously.

Contributing to the Community

We as Americans have a long history of contributing to the community. From the barn-raisings of colonial times to today's more formal volunteering programs, we've long known how important it is to help others.

These days, there are plenty of opportunities to help. You can work with animals; with children, teens, or adults; or by yourself. You can take on a public role or operate behind the scenes. You can volunteer daily, weekly, monthly, or sporadically—whatever fits into your schedule. And you know that everything you do, be it stuffing envelopes or delivering food, is something that wouldn't happen without you.

Although we've always realized that it is important that we all contribute to the community, we haven't always been aware of how volunteer work helps with our own physical and mental health.

Leading medical research has shown that states with high levels of volunteerism have lower rates of mortality and heart disease. According to the Corporation for National and Community Service, people who volunteer regularly not only help their communities, but also experience better health as they get older in terms of having higher functional ability, lower rates of depression, and overall greater longevity. Community involvement can also help you keep physically fit.

In addition, volunteering offers many benefits in terms of mental health. Contributing to the community aids in the following ways:

- Feeling a sense of belonging in the community
- Enhancing social networks
- Contributing to a sense of purpose
- Building connections, both personal and professional
- Developing professional skills
- Increasing social and relationship skills
- Protecting against isolation and loneliness
- Developing self-confidence
- Improving overall life satisfaction

Important Points

- Having a positive attitude can improve heart health.
- Negative emotions can hurt heart health.
- Negative emotions include depression, anger/hostility, anxiety, social isolation, and stress.

- After a heart-disease diagnosis, many people experience emotional concerns.
- These postdiagnosis issues can make it harder to adopt a heart-healthy lifestyle—and can increase the risk of bad outcomes.
- Volunteering is not only good for the community, but it is good for your physical and mental health.

CHAPTER 10
Spirituality and Meditation

AS WE'VE SEEN, THE FIGHT-OR-FLIGHT instinct is vital to human preservation and harmful to the human heart muscle. So what's the alternative?

According to Herbert Benson, MD, director emeritus of the Benson-Henry Institute for Mind/Body Medicine, it is the relaxation response, a physiologic state of deep rest that you can achieve through practices such as meditation and prayer. He adds that this state produces immediate changes in the expression of genes involved in immune function, energy metabolism, and insulin secretion.

Spiritual practices, such as prayer, meditation, and tai chi, can have an effect on medical patients of all sorts, notably heart patients.

Leading medical research suggests that spirituality can reduce depression, improve blood pressure, and boost the immune system. Religious beliefs and practices can help patients fight feelings of helplessness, restore meaning and order to life situations, and promote regaining a sense of control. Spirituality can be a powerful and important source of strength.

Contemplative Practices

Medical research suggest that regular contemplative practice that provides heart health benefits. These sorts of practices guide those who do them to focus their attention in a specific way. Often, people concentrate on reflecting inward or on a specific sensation or concept.

Please remember that none of these approaches are replacements for proper medical care. Try spirituality and meditation *in addition* to seeing your doctor and following any prescribed medical regimen.

Prayer

Prayer can help people relax and think about hope, gratitude, and compassion. It can provide a sense of comfort, connection, and well-being. Sometimes it can help people feel that there is a benevolent force out there that cares about them.

Prayer can give patients a sense of hope and optimism and a reduced feeling of powerlessness. Leading medical research also indicates that prayer can lead to fewer medical complications; lowered blood pressure and heart rate; decreased mortality from coronary heart disease; a higher survival rate following cardiac surgery; and improved postsurgical recovery, including wound appearance, lower fever, and less pain.

Another component of spiritual practice that can be helpful is the idea of forgiveness. Letting go of negative feelings can be beneficial. Leading medical research suggests that forgiveness can improve immune function, extend the life-span, lower blood pressure, improve overall cardiovascular health, and lead to fewer feelings of anger or hurt. It can also improve quality of life.

Meditation

Meditation helps you let go of stress and feel peaceful and relaxed. According to the American Heart Association, meditation can lower your blood pressure, improve the quality of your sleep, reduce anxiety and depression, and lower your risk of heart disease. It can also produce feelings of calmness and clearheadedness and can improve your ability to concentrate and feel compassion.

There are many types of meditation practices, but according to the National Center for Complementary and Alternative Medicine (NCCAM), they all have four elements in common:

+ A quiet setting with as few distractions as possible
+ A specific, comfortable posture (such as sitting, lying down, or walking)

- A focus of attention (a specially chosen word or set of words, an object, or the sensations of the breath)
- A nonjudgmental attitude (allowing distractions to appear without judging them)

Studies suggest that meditation can reduce blood pressure, ease anxiety and depression, and help with insomnia.

We will focus on mindfulness-based stress reduction (MBSR), which was developed specifically to help people facing serious illness, and transcendental meditation (TM), which has been studied for its effects on medical patients and is the only type of meditation supported by the American Heart Association.

Mindfulness-Based Stress Reduction

MBSR was developed by Jon Kabat-Zinn at the University of Massachusetts Medical School specifically to teach participants to cope with stress, pain, and illness. The practice is about taking control of your life, being aware of things that affect your well-being and health, and finding peace of mind and balance. Not only was it started in a medical facility, but it is now offered in more than two hundred medical centers, offices, and clinics.

As Kabat-Zinn suggests, MBSR is the emotional equivalent of weather preparedness for sailors. Sailors try to avoid being at sea during a bad storm, but if they are, they know how to cope. Similarly, MBSR cannot help you avoid all of the challenges of life, but it can help you steer through them safely.

In general, MBSR is seen as decreasing depression, anxiety, and stress and improving overall psychological health. It can also be helpful in pain management.

When done traditionally, MBSR is an eight-week workshop taught by certified trainers. Participants meet weekly for instruction and practice and have homework that typically involves daily meditation. MBSR uses three formal techniques: mindfulness meditation (focusing on a single object or subject), body scanning (focusing on the body from head to toes, one part at a time), and simple yoga postures. The goal is to develop an awareness of moment-to-moment experiences.

Transcendental Meditation

TM is a technique for promoting relaxed awareness. Typically, you practice TM by sitting in a comfortable position, eyes closed, and silently repeat a mantra (a meaningless sound that has been assigned to you). It requires no concentration or monitoring of thoughts. To learn TM, you must work one-on-one with a certified instructor.

According to the official TM website, the practice offers the following benefits:

+ Increased inner calm
+ Reduced cortisol
+ Improved blood pressure
+ Reduced insomnia
+ Decreased risk of heart attack and stroke
+ Lower levels of anxiety and depression
+ Improved brain function and memory

According to the American Heart Association, TM is the only meditation practice that has been shown to lower blood pressure. But it's unclear whether other forms of meditation are less effective, or have just been studied less thoroughly.

Tai Chi

Sometimes called "moving meditation," tai chi has been shown to improve the quality of life for heart patients, according to the NCCAM. Specifically, it can improve the following:

+ Exercise capacity
+ Quality of life
+ Physical activity
+ Mood

Tai chi, which originated in China as a martial art, is another mind-body practice. It is a noncompetitive, self-paced system of gentle physical exercise and stretching, with a focus on deep breathing and posture. Each position flows into the next without pause, so you are in constant motion. People practice tai chi individually or in groups.

Although it started as a martial art, tai chi is very gentle. You can practice it even if you're not in great shape or in perfect health. A typical tai chi class has three components:

+ **Warm-up**: Involves easy motions designed to loosen your muscles and joints and start your focus on breathing.
+ **Instruction**: Involves the practice of shorter and longer forms, depending on the style of tai chi. Practitioners recommend starting with shorter forms because they have smaller and slower movements.
+ **Quigong**: Means breath work or energy work and involves a few minutes of gentle breathing designed to relax the mind and mobilize your energy.

There is no certification for teachers of tai chi, so you might want to chat with an instructor about his or her training and experience before signing up.

Leading medical research has found that tai chi offers several benefits to heart patients:

+ Boosts exercise capacity
+ Lowers blood pressure
+ Improves levels of cholesterol, insulin, and C-reactive protein
+ Decreases triglyceride level

Practicing tai chi helps you cultivate energy for your body, mind, and spirit. You can apply this newfound energy to everything you do.

Millions of Americans use some form of complementary and alternative medicine (CAM). But this type of treatment is meant to be used in conjunction with traditional medical care. Don't turn to prayer, meditation, or tai chi instead of conventional medical treatment or even as a reason to delay seeking medical help. These approaches are meant to provide additional support and comfort and added health benefits, not a cure. That's why they're called "complementary."

Important Points

- Complementary approaches can aid in heart healthnotably spirituality, meditation, and tai chi.
- Spirituality can offer a sense of hope and optimism, which is good for your heart.
- There are many types of meditation, so you can find what works best for you. Two of the most popular are MBSR and TM.
- MBSR was designed by a medical doctor specifically to help people with chronic or serious medical conditions.
- TM is probably the most studied form of meditation from a medical perspective and offers documented benefits to the heart.
- Tai chi is a form of "moving meditation" that has been shown to help heart patients in several ways.
- Prayer, meditation, and tai chi are meant to supplement traditional medical care, not replace it.

CHAPTER 11

Conclusion

AS WE'VE SEEN, HEART DISEASE is a scary thing. It's the number-one cause of death in the United States and around the world, and it accounts for more than a third of a million American deaths every year. When you add in the risk of stroke and other cardiovascular diseases, the figure more than doubles.

We've also discussed the risk factors that you're just stuck with. You can't change your age, gender, race, and family history—and all contribute to the possibility of heart disease.

Fortunately, there's actually quite a bit you can do to improve your heart health and stave off heart disease. It mostly comes down to making lifestyle changes.

First, though, you have to take charge of your heart health. You must decide that you want to improve the physical condition of that precious fist-sized muscle. Making this decision is critical; it's easier, of course, just to ignore warning signs and have that extra bowl of ice cream, watch that extra hour of television, skip going to the gym, or have one more drink. But if you want to improve your quality of life and longevity, you have to first decide to take action.

The next step is to figure out what your personal risk factors are. It's hard to know what sorts of positive changes to make in your daily life if you don't know where you need that extra little nudge of healthful behavior. This book outlines the risk factors, and that can be a good place to start.

You should also discuss the issue with your doctor when you have your annual physical exam. Your doctor will conduct a series of screenings and early detection tests that will indicate what you can do to improve your heart health.

Things to Think About

First, think about your level of physical activity. Your heart is a muscle. And like any other muscle, it needs exercise to stay strong. Chapter 6 outlines the amount and types of exercise that are most helpful to improving heart health. Remember, though, to have fun while you exercise. Just because your best friend loves tennis doesn't mean that you're up for a one-on-one competition; you might prefer jogging or taking a belly-dancing class. Think about what *you* enjoy because, if it's fun, you're more likely to stick with it.

Another key element to heart health is nutrition. Just as we put the best fuel into our cars, we need to feed our bodies with the best possible food for the best possible results. Chapter 7 outlines the types of foods that are heart healthy and pointed out the types of items and preparation approaches to avoid. With a little effort, you can have heart-healthy food that's just as yummy for you as what you may have been eating before. And you'll feel much better afterward, as will your heart.

Weight control is also important. Not only does your body need the right types of food, it also needs the right amount. When you're fueling your car, the gas pump will click off when the tank is full. Unfortunately, our stomachs don't have a similar mechanism. We need to watch our portion sizes—as they relate to the energy we expend—to make sure that our body mass index (BMI) is in the healthy range.

Sleep is a difficult issue in this day and age when everything and everybody seems to operate 24-7. But while computers and machines can do that without problems, our bodies need regular sleep, and plenty of it, on a nightly basis. Chapter 8 details the amount of sleep necessary at each life stage. When you get enough sleep, you not only improve your heart health, but you also feel better day to day.

Another issue—and one that is often harder to control—is your emotions. Studies have shown that depression, anxiety, anger, and loneliness all take a toll on the human heart—and more than you might have realized. Fortunately, there is much you can do to improve the situation. Chapter 9 discusses specific suggestions. But the overarching issue here is to relax and enjoy life. Why worry so much about longevity if each day is a slog? Relax, spend time with others, and enjoy yourself. It's some of the best medicine possible.

In chapter 10, we outline some additional approaches that can help improve your heart health. Spirituality, meditation, and tai chi are all options in your heart-health toolbox that can improve your quality of life and heart health.

Although the issue of heart health can be scary, it can also be exhilarating. There is so much we can do to improve our situations and our health. All we need to do is reach out and take those opportunities in order to take control of our own life—and enjoy it.

ABOUT THE AUTHOR

EARNING HIS MEDICAL DEGREE FROM the University of Cairo, Egypt, Dr. Shalaby completed his Internal Medicine residency at the University of Missouri, Columbia and a cardiology fellowship training in the world-renowned Ochsner Clinic Foundation in New Orleans - where he worked under the direction of the nation's most esteemed cardiologists.

Dr. Shalaby is board certified in Cardiovascular Disease - and a member of prestigious cardiology and scientific associations. He is also a Fellow of the American College of Cardiology.

Practicing a range of cardiovascular medicine with special interest in new technologies in cardiac imaging, including cardiac CT and cardiac MRI, Dr. Shalaby obtained specialized training in peripheral vascular disease diagnosis and management.

His comprehensive experience with early detection of cardiac disease and preventive Cardiology has enabled him to design multiple cardiac wellness and preventive programs that employ education, diet, exercise, behavioral therapy and life style modifications to prevent and reduce the severity of heart disease.

Dr. Shalaby's work in early detection, weight reduction and fitness programs is saving lives of many and has changed the lives of many of his patients and friends.

A truly dedicated professional, Dr. Shalaby is a staff cardiologist at the Texas Heart Institute, the St. Luke Hospital, Clear Lake Regional Medical Center, Memorial South East Hospital, St. John Hospital and the Mainland Medical Center.

He lectures at the local and national level on the early detection of heart disease, weight loss and cardiac disease, exercise and wellness programs and a wide variety of cardiac health-related topics.

Printed in the United States
By Bookmasters